Pain and Profits

BOOKSTORE
USED

Pain and Profits

The History of the Headache and Its Remedies in America

JAN R. MCTAVISH

RUTGERS UNIVERSITY PRESS

NEW BRUNSWICK, NEW JERSEY, AND LONDON

LIBRARY OF CONGRESS CATALOGING-IN-PUBLICATION DATA

McTavish, Janice Rae.
    Pain and profits : the history of the headache and its remedies in America /
Jan R. McTavish.
        p.   cm.
    Includes bibliographical references and index.
    ISBN 0-8135-3440-2 (hbk. : alk. paper) — ISBN 0-8135-3441-0 (pbk. : alk. paper)
    I. Headache.   2. Headache—Treatment—History.   I. Title.
    RB128.M386 2004
    616.8'49106—dc22   2003022265

British Cataloging-in-Publication information for this book is available
from the British Library.

Copyright © 2004 by Jan R. McTavish

All rights reserved

No part of this book may be reproduced or utilized in any form or by any means,
electronic or mechanical, or by any information storage and retrieval system,
without written permission from the publisher. Please contact Rutgers University
Press, 100 Joyce Kilmer Avenue, Piscataway, NJ 08854–8099. The only exception to
this prohibition is "fair use" as defined by U.S. copyright law.

Manufactured in the United States of America

CONTENTS

ACKNOWLEDGMENTS

So many individuals and organizations have helped me in my research on painkillers, aspirin, headaches, and the drug industry, and so many years have passed since I began this work in graduate school, nursing parts of it through term papers at the University of Toronto, a master's thesis on aspirin at the University of Minnesota, and a dissertation on headache at York University, that I am afraid I cannot possibly name everyone who provided scholarly, financial, or moral support. So I apologize in advance to those whose names do not appear here, but be assured that your assistance was greatly appreciated and extremely useful. I could not have done it without you. All errors of fact, of course, and all misinterpretations are my own.

My thanks therefore to University of Toronto classmate Sandy McRae; University of Minnesota faculty John Eyler and Mary Jo Maynes, History of Medicine secretary Kathy Kosiak, former Wangensteen Historical Library staff Judith Overmier and Cheryl Owens; Hans-Hermann Pogarell of the Bayer Unternehmensarchiv, Leverkusen; the staffs of the American Pharmaceutical Association, the Consumer Healthcare Products Association, the National Library of Medicine, all in Washington, D.C.; the staff of the libraries at the University of Toronto, York University, and the University of Winnipeg; York University dissertation supervisor Richard Jarrell; Gregory Higby and Elaine Stroud of the American Institute of the History of Pharmacy, the Sonnedecker Residency fund for the History of Pharmacy, University of Wisconsin; the Hannah Institute for the History of Medicine, for a Grant-in-Aid; Alcorn State University, for an Intellectual Renewal Grant; John Swann, historian of the Food and Drug Administration; the staff at the National Archives, Washington, D.C.; Thomas Reimer; Charles Rosenberg who read the original manuscript; Audra Wolfe and Adi Hovav at Rutgers University Press; Theresa and Lonnie Schenck, Suzanne LeMay-Sheffield, Darlene Abreu-Ferreira, Karen Johnson, and last but not least, Ian.

Pain and Profits

Introduction

Thomas Jefferson used to get headaches. He did not get them very often—only once every ten years or so—but what they lacked in frequency they made up for in severity. Later in life he described the pain as excruciating, and we know that he suffered for days at a time, sometimes for weeks. These headaches incapacitated him and must have been a serious disruption in his busy life. Yet in his letters to his family he did little more than mention that he had "had an attack." He did not provide many details: perhaps his family was already so familiar with the situation that he did not need to elaborate. At any rate, Jefferson seems to have been resigned to his affliction and did not bemoan his fate.[1] In his stoicism, he is typical of his era. Indeed, if we did not have medical literature to tell us otherwise, we might suppose that headaches were altogether rare events in the eighteenth and nineteenth centuries, so uncommon and so unenlightening are the references to them. But tucked away in footnotes and memoranda, in marginalia and perfunctory comments to friends and relatives, the headache is in fact revealed as an omnipresent and unpleasant condition, as common then as it is today. The only major difference is that Americans of earlier times simply did not complain much about them. Had they done so, however, they would have found an audience far more sympathetic than usually exists today. Although it was not thought to be as serious as so many of the other health problems of those days, the headache was nevertheless taken seriously. It was as real and as wretched as a toothache. No one accused Jefferson of pretending or exaggerating in order to avoid an obligation.[2] When he said he had a bad headache, his friends and family believed him and sympathized.

By the twenty-first century, however, the situation had become somewhat different. Soon after World War I, the headache was at once more conspicuous and more ignominious. It began to be referred to casually in literature, in the movies, and eventually television. People now seem to grumble about their headaches all the time. In the United States alone there are said to be 45 million chronic sufferers (whose headaches occur more than fifteen days a month), and 25 to 30 million with migraines. Countless millions more have headaches only once in awhile but suffer enough to take time off work or to cancel a social engagement. Moreover, the word now has an additional meaning. Dwight D. Eisenhower, for example, had ileitis, bursitis, arthritis, and a couple of heart attacks, but the headaches he referred to in his diary were a wartime supply problem ("Ships! Ships! All we need is ships! . . . What a headache!") and a cold war diplomatic difficulty ("Monday I go to Turkey and Greece. More headaches and problems.").[3] By the 1920s or thereabouts, the word *headache* had slipped into the American vernacular to refer to "something, such as a problem, that causes annoyance or trouble."[4] The headache is now just a "pain in the neck," so to speak.

At about the same time, medical headaches began to be viewed with less sympathy and more suspicion, seen not as legitimate ailments but as the domain of whiners, malingerers, neurotics, and especially of frigid women. "Not tonight, dear, I've got a headache" has become a kind of mantra of the modern dysfunctional marriage. Consider John Steinbeck's pitiless description of Mrs. Bernice Pritchard in *The Wayward Bus*, published in 1948. She hated sex and resented her husband's advances, so to punish him she used headaches that were so bad "they twisted her face and reduced her to a panting, sweating, grinning, quivering blob of pain." She also used them to control her daughter. Steinbeck implies that Bernice either faked these migraines or deliberately conjured them but that in any case they were not quite "real." The daughter, at least, did not believe them. Her mother needed a psychiatrist, she thought, not a neurologist.[5] Bernice is an invented character, of course, but Steinbeck's attitude toward her headaches reflects more than his personal point of view or that of the general public. It also represents a position held at midcentury by many in the medical profession. By the 1950s, major and minor headaches alike were being described as the result of an inability to deal with the "resentments and dissatisfactions" that were a part of everyday life. People who got headaches brought them on themselves. The pain was real (although there were sometimes doubts even about this), but the solution was to learn to relax, or "grow up," or not be so self-centered. It was only a headache, after all. It would go away on its own.

In the 150 years between Jefferson and Steinbeck, the headache appears to have undergone a transformation, devolving from a respectable complaint into a somewhat disreputable cliché. But why did this happen? And why should anyone, least of all a historian, care? Headaches are hardly comparable to cancer or tuberculosis. They are certainly unpleasant; occasionally (as in brain tumors) they warn of a fatal outcome, and they have sometimes driven people to suicide, but in themselves they are not considered dangerous.

Yet headaches do in fact possess both medical and historical significance. As common, painful complaints encountered by all practitioners, they allow us a glimpse into the mundane medical events that most physicians had to deal with most of the time. They also demonstrate the challenges that "ordinary" ailments posed and can tell us something about medical imagination and innovation when faced with an ailment that, on the one hand, was run-of-the-mill but on the other was frustratingly protean. The only feature all headaches share, as it turns out, is the "ache." Beyond that, the pain can take myriad forms. It can be of any intensity, it can be located in any part of the head, occur at any interval, last for any length of time. Some headaches appear to be triggered by chocolate, others by fatigue, alcohol, sunshine, or a disagreeable smell. Any disease at all can be made infinitely more miserable by the presence of a headache, but they also occur on their own, spontaneously, without obvious precipitating factors. Their one virtue is that the majority are transient. Indeed, most are only moderately painful, short-lived, and occasional. Their variety, in fact, has meant that with the possible exception of migraine, a headache has never been considered to be a disease in itself: it has always been a symptom, a clue only, a sign of some deeper dysfunction. For much of the nineteenth century, at least, this ensured that headaches were never irrelevant. In a medical philosophy derived from a holistic, constitutional, and often humoral view of disease, visible or reported symptoms of all kinds were invaluable diagnostic tools. The complicated art of interpreting these signs gave the physician an opportunity to exercise his particular skills and knowledge. As a prominent if perplexing symptom with many manifestations, the headache fit quite comfortably into this system. But this also meant that physicians were not inclined to use analgesics to treat it, because the goal of therapy was to get rid of the cause of the pain rather than the pain itself. Painkillers—that is, the opiates—were usually considered inappropriate.

By the early years of the twentieth century, advances in science had created an environment in which medical ideas were increasingly based on physical evidence—bacteria, blood pressure measurements, blood chemistry, and so on, supported by new diagnostic techniques. X-rays, for example, could now substantiate that in many painful conditions there was indeed something physically wrong with the part that hurt. Unfortunately, headaches produced no such visible or measurable features. They exhibited no tissue damage, no bruises, no bumps; they left no scars in the cranium, on the brain, or anywhere else. They were singularly uncooperative when it came to revealing why they hurt. Yet also around the turn of the century, advances in pharmaceutical chemistry introduced several new drugs such as aspirin that proved to be effective and relatively safe painkillers and became very popular as headache remedies—without shedding any light on the pathology of the headache or increasing the medical profession's understanding of the phenomenon. But because these new drugs could (and did) alleviate most ordinary headaches fairly quickly, in the twentieth century the headache was no longer a challenging piece of a diagnostic puzzle but simply an inconvenient and unpleasant experience for the patient and an annoying distraction for the doctor. Although not exactly thought to be irrelevant, the headache was now a "bother," just as many other inconvenient and unpleasant but not serious problems were now "headaches." Severe or chronic headaches, on the other hand, lacking physical confirmation of their existence and usually unaffected by the new drugs, now entered the realm of psychological disorders, and their sufferers began to be labeled as neurotic: "It's all in your head." Not surprisingly, headache victims did not always appreciate this attitude.

The headache therefore also provides an opportunity to explore many other important features of American medicine as it developed in the last century and a half. It tells us something, for instance, about the evolution of the relationship between physicians and the laity in a world of rapidly changing medical ideas, of scientific advances, and increasing professionalization. The headache lets us know that despite the growing authority of physicians and their increasingly abstruse, science-based explanations of disease and ill health, patients nevertheless retained significant control over their medical affairs, seeking or ignoring doctors' advice as it suited them. American traditions of self-care were in fact reinforced by experiences with the headache. Often dissatisfied with professional treatment, patients chose other options.

But much of what we know about headaches in the nineteenth and even in the twentieth century comes not from patients, nor from clinical notes or patient files that may lie yet undiscovered in archives and attics, but from the published writings of medical professionals, a fact that necessarily limits our perspective. There is, however, another fertile source of information about headaches, one that not only allows us to extrapolate more of the patient's point of view but that also enriches our understanding of professional medicine and—most importantly—provides an avenue into an area of medical history that scholars often overlook: drug supply. Doctors' reluctance to treat headaches with analgesics in the nineteenth century did not mean that the headache was not treated. Indeed, the ubiquity and variety of its appearances meant that headache remedies were numerous and inventive, and that full use was made of a therapeutic repertoire, both lay and professional, that stretched back to ancient times. Almost all such treatments made extensive use of drugs. Historians do not often question how drugs, medicinal preparations, and pharmaceutical chemicals became available, but given that they were as essential in nineteenth- and early twentieth-century medical practices as they are today, pharmaceutical manufacturers, the drug trade, and the profession of pharmacy deserve our attention. Until recently, however, it has simply been assumed that the products of modern pharmaceutical science that began to emerge about a hundred years ago have always been largely in the control of the medical profession, for good or ill.

The story of headache remedies—and most particularly, of the German synthetic remedies such as Aspirin introduced in the last two decades of the nineteenth century—demonstrates that the drug trade had a far more vital and active role than is sometimes acknowledged. Profitability, marketing concerns, and property laws could be just as critical to a drug's use as its efficacy or safety. The relationship between physicians and pharmaceutical manufacturers was thus of particular concern to medical reformers in the late nineteenth and early twentieth centuries, who were worried that American doctors were poorly educated in the complexities of drug use and prescribing. They feared that drug makers' advertising and promotional materials were becoming substitutes for proper training. And they objected to the increasing presence of commercial enterprises in what was supposed to be the altruistic principles of professional, scientific practice. It was an unconscionable intrusion of mercenary notions into humanitarian concerns. The headache remedies are a particularly good example of this interplay, selling for millions, then billions of dollars by the end of the twentieth century.

Another topic of interest—and again, a concern to medical reformers—was the drug industry's eventual targeting of the public, not just doctors, as the best market for its headache treatments. Before the middle of the nineteenth century, drug makers had made no real distinctions between the professional and the lay markets, but as medical practice became more scientific and exclusive, some manufacturers, in an effort to be seen as equal in altruism and erudition to physicians, evolved into a branch of the industry known as "ethical." Although the term obviously was intended to have positive connotations, it really meant (and was viewed at the time to mean) that regardless of what other behavior it might engage in, such a company did not advertise its wares to the public and was thus proudly superior to the nostrum or proprietary drug firms whose primary target was every American man, woman, and child.

Pink Pills for Pale People, Hamlin's Wizard Oil, Lydia Pinkham's Vegetable Compound, and a host of other famous and infamous concoctions trumpeted their goods as guaranteed remedies for every conceivable ailment, life-threatening or merely irksome. So it is not surprising that when the painkilling synthetic drugs were invented, the patent medicine companies began to market them as headache remedies to a population hungry for such relief. But in fact it was not the nostrum makers who brought this property to the attention of the public. The public had discovered it for themselves; nostrum makers simply followed the public's lead. So too did some ethical firms, attracted by the potential for huge profits that direct public sales could mean. The Bayer Company's handling of its Phenacetin and Aspirin (both of which it invented and introduced as ethical products) is a particularly good example of this process and allows us to examine how both the public and the manufacturers influenced the medical environment, despite the growing efforts of the medical profession to discourage self-treatment and rein in the excesses of the drug trade. The history of the headache and its remedies in fact is a kind of counterexample to the general notion that with the advent of modern medicine, American doctors became all-powerful (whether this is seen as a good thing or not). Indeed, by the end of World War I, some of the most highly respected state-of-the-art medications available were very clearly not in the charge of physicians.

The inability of the American medical profession to gain control of nonnarcotic analgesics such as aspirin is ironic. The drugs, after all, demonstrated the potential that nineteenth-century chemistry had for improving medical practice and enhancing its prestige—exactly the sort of result that the profession had hoped for from the new medical sciences. That the doctors in a sense lost the opportunity to be the sole guardians of drugs that were not only models of scientific achievement but also keenly appreciated by the public suggests that physicians were neither the authoritative and learned profession they thought they were nor the monolithic and imperious brotherhood claimed by their critics. Also ironic is the fact that although the new drugs proved to be very good at handling many headaches, those unfortunate persons for whom the drugs were not effective now faced not only a skeptical medical profession but also often friends and family unsympathetic to their plight. Only since the 1960s has the American medical profession again begun to pay as much attention to the headache as a medical problem as well as a psychological one, but what this will mean for the headache in the twenty-first century remains to be seen.

The history of the headache in the United States in the last 150 years shows that this ailment had a small but lively role in helping to establish, shape, and sustain the various jurisdictions and relationships among the medical professions, pharmaceutical interests, and the public at large, leading to the creation of the modern headache remedy industry and to the headache as simply another "headache" common to modern life.

1

The Headache and Its Treatment in the Nineteenth Century

On the sunny spring morning of 9 April 1865, a few miles west of the small Virginia town of Appomattox Court House, General Ulysses S. Grant, commander of the Union forces, was in no mood to admire the weather. He had some urgent problems facing him, including the troubling uncertainty of Robert E. Lee's next move. Would Lee fight? The remnants of the Army of Northern Virginia had escaped from Petersburg and were heading toward a defensible position at Lynchburg, where it was expected they would make a gallant, if ultimately futile, last stand. But the Union infantry under General Phil Sheridan had moved faster than even the North's leaders had anticipated and in fact had cut Lee off before he reached his destination. With the Confederates outnumbered and surrounded at Appomattox, the eventual outcome was never in question, but the rebels were scrappy, and the casualties on both sides would be high. Grant was determined that it would not be he who made the first move. He did not want to be responsible for a bloodbath this late in the war. He sent notes across the line to Lee, but Lee's responses were not encouraging. Grant fretted, his mood made all the worse by the fact that he had not slept well the night before. Indeed, Grant's other urgent problem that morning was a very painful sick headache. It had come on him the previous afternoon, stayed with him all night, and still tormented him hours later.

A tough, experienced soldier accustomed to the discomfort of campaigns and the rigors of military life, Grant recorded few illnesses of any kind during his years in the army. He had suffered occasional painful conditions, however, such as toothache or leg cramps, and once, when his horse fell on him, injuring his leg, "the pain was almost beyond endurance." He also recorded several bad headaches, for which on at least one occasion he took "medicine"—very likely a narcotic. His remark to his wife about "those terrible headaches which you know I am subject to" suggests he experienced the affliction even more often than his diary mentions. We can be reasonably sure, then, that his Appomattox headache was a very unpleasant experience. Even Grant's staff was well aware of his condition and unsettled by it. Unfortunately, the general's attempts to get rid of the headache by means of hot mustard foot baths and mustard plasters applied to his wrists and neck had proved futile. He could have used laudanum (tincture of opium), but it seems he avoided narcotics this time, probably because they would have clouded his mind. But at ten minutes before noon, still "suffering severely," Grant received a message from Lee that resolved both of his difficulties in one fell swoop. Lee was prepared to surrender: "The instant I saw the contents of the note I was cured."[1] The headache vanished.

A few months later, and a few hundred miles farther south in Camden, South Carolina—a town Grant's colleague General Sherman had burned in February—Mary Boykin Chesnut was not so lucky. There was no good news to cure the headache she had on 4 July 1865 ("one of my worst"), and in fact it forced her to stay in bed all day. A woman of great passion, intelligence, wit, and charm, Chesnut had been born to a life of privilege and comfort in the antebellum South but now struggled to deal with the bewildering change in her circumstances. Her diary of her Civil War experiences provides rich details of those times—the stress, deprivations, and the occasional small comforts. Although in general she faced her trials courageously, she also suffered from frequent spells of anxiety and depression that made her ill. One could be forgiven for thinking that Mrs. Chesnut—a Confederate aristocrat and a flower of southern womanhood, after all—might simply have been having a case of "the vapors." She was watching her world disintegrate around her. That she should occasionally have taken refuge in illness is not so unreasonable. But those who read her journal know she was made of sterner stuff. She suffered from angina, and most if not all of her bouts of ill health appear to be genuine. The pain was at times intense enough for her to resort to opium—a drug she revered for its power to soothe her, but it also left her somewhat befuddled, and she suspected it would eventually contribute to her death. Interspersed with her angina attacks, too, were other less threatening but nonetheless troublesome conditions—"neuralgia of the eyes," "congestion of the lungs"— and headaches. Chesnut, like Grant, recorded her headaches on only a few occasions, although she too implies that she got them rather more often. How she tried to get rid of them, however, she does not say. Certainly the opium and morphine she took for her angina—the only real painkillers available at that time—were never mentioned in connection with her headaches. She appears simply to have gone to her room and waited them out. In Mary Chesnut's world, a headache was the least of her problems.[2]

For both Chesnut and Grant, headaches were unwelcome and unpleasant but of less concern to them than other aspects of their health. In this, they are typical of their fellow citizens. Americans did not describe their headaches in detail and did not often bother to record what they did to get rid of them. Even Thomas Jefferson's terrible headaches rated nothing more than the acknowledgment of their existence and his plaintively expressed hope that they would eventually go away. If he took any medicines to hasten their departure, he does not tell us. Chesnut's angina, and Grant's fatal cancer in 1885, on the other hand, both excruciating, understandably received far more attention from their sufferers. Clearly a headache paled in comparison. But even people who were preoccupied, almost obsessed, with all facets of their own ill health, describing their afflictions in lurid, loving detail, mentioned headache only infrequently. Alice James, sister of Henry and William, suffered from a life of "nervous prostration" yet made only indirect reference to the headaches that accompanied this condition.[3] Her brother Henry likewise discussed a number of ailments that in his younger days included a particularly vicious kind of constipation, but he only referred obliquely to his head being "all out of order."[4] The chronically indisposed Emily Dickinson does not seem to have mentioned the word. Louisa May Alcott considered herself permanently invalided after her stint in an army hospital in 1862, but headache was not usually what plagued her, although in early 1887 she did admit that her "head does ache a good deal" and that it affected her mood.[5] Metaphorical headaches are also absent, and only Henry James came close when his American in Paris "sat down with an aesthetic headache" because "his attention had been strained and his eyes dazzled" by an art exhibit.[6] Fictional characters, too, who succumbed to consumption, pneumonia, scarlet fever, typhoid, or vague, unspecified, and romantic afflictions may also have suffered from some sort of "nervous weakness," but they rarely seemed to get headaches. At least, like their real counterparts, they did not mention them very often.

This relative absence of headaches—especially of the ordinary, garden-variety kind—from the pages of diaries, letters, and fiction could mean that Americans of the nineteenth century in fact did not get headaches very often. Or that they simply did not complain about them very much. The evidence overwhelmingly supports the latter conclusion. There are enough "between-the-lines" references to head pain to suggest that all classes, races, ages, and both sexes endured headaches just as frequently then as they do today. Medical writings in fact substantiate this by explicitly noting how common the "common headache" really was. "Vast numbers [of headache victims] are submitting patiently to it everywhere," observed one sympathetic practitioner in 1870.[7] But it seems that people just did not grumble publicly about something so generally insignificant, especially when measured against the other afflictions from which one might suffer. In a collection of diaries of pioneer women whose hardships were legion (cholera, typhus, snakebite, diarrhea, accidents), there was apparently only one report of a headache: on 24 May 1853, Amelia Stewart Knight, mother of seven children and pregnant with the eighth, heading west to Oregon from Iowa, recorded: "I had the sick headache all night, some better this morning; must do a day's work."[8]

In Protestant America, pain was part of God's plan, often regarded as fitting punishment for sin or as a test of faith. It would have been impious to protest against it. If nothing else, it built character. Pain was seen as an unavoidable, perhaps necessary, fact of life.[9] And when Americans did discuss their painful disorders, the descriptions are usually of such terrible or grave conditions that it is difficult to believe that any headache but the most debilitating migraine could measure up. With the opiates the only real painkillers available, Americans were judicious in selecting what to complain about. The narcotics were too precious to be used just because something hurt. It had to hurt a lot. Mary Chesnut, for instance, suffering one of her angina attacks, described the friend who brought her opium—

scarce, because of the war—as an "angel." And General Grant, dying of throat cancer in 1885, relied heavily on morphine to give him some respite, showing real fear when he discovered that it was beginning to lose its power. No wonder people were reluctant to use these drugs for a mere headache. And no wonder headaches were low on the scale of complaints, given the numbers of men, women, and children who, like Grant and Chesnut, faced agonizing and often fatal diseases.

Although Americans may have suffered their headaches silently, they did not necessarily suffer them passively. Transient and occasional, the headache was an appropriate malady for treating at home; many of the allusions to its omnipresence in American life come from the lists of remedies in domestic medical literature. In some ways, Americans were fortunate when it came to home care, because as inhabitants of a nation populated by people from various cultures, they had the opportunity to consult the entire world's accumulated wisdom on headaches. Not only could Americans draw on the ancient, classical notions of professional physicians; they also had access to the household healing traditions of the English-speaking world as well as those of other European immigrants, indigenous peoples, and African slaves. A headache sufferer was never very far from some remedy or other.

A significant portion of these home remedies was essentially magical. Every ethnic or regional group had its favorite customs whose origins were lost in time but that shared a number of features common to this style of healing. Some methods were based on morbid associations—always a powerful facet of the occult. Pennsylvania folk wisdom, for example, suggested that the headache sufferer tie a bit of rope from a hangman's noose (preferably one that had been used) around her head. Many other folk treatments similarly relied on the principle that things associated with the head must be good for a headache: snuff made from moss growing inside a human skull and potions made from plants growing on the head of a statue were thought to be effective. So were strategies that attempted to transfer the headache from the sufferer to some other creature or object. In the Bahamas the descendants of slaves were said to have carefully tied two live frogs to the temples of a headache victim, leaving them there until the creatures were all but dead. After the animals were freed, they were expected to die quickly, the headache dying with them. The amphibians must have objected, so this technique may not have been very popular—certainly not with frogs—and does not seem to have been imported to the United States itself. In North Carolina, on the other hand, although frogs might be spared, other animals were not: a mole could be pressed (literally) into service. Someone who had squeezed a mole to death was believed to be able to cure headache by touch, using the hand that had done the deed. An even more widespread practice was based on the belief that headache was caused by the evil eye and therefore could be prevented (although not cured, apparently) by means of prayers, incantations, and amulets.[10] Yet despite the fact that magical solutions could draw on the infinite resources of the occult, it is perhaps surprising that the repertoire contained relatively few treatments directed specifically at headaches. This could mean, of course, that the mole-cure or the rope-cure worked very well and that no other course of action was needed. Or it could mean that supernatural forces were not to be squandered any more than earthly resources were for something as insignificant as the average headache. More serious ailments such as whooping cough, croup, and—overwhelmingly—warts got far more attention. (Warts were visible and ugly, and no doubt questions of vanity were involved.)

As for more "commonsense" folk remedies, the first and likely the most common way to treat a headache (as opposed to simply ignoring it) was with a local or topical application, based on the self-evident notion that the site of the pain should be the site of the treatment. Such remedies might consist of a cloth dampened with water and perhaps some additional soothing substance such as lavender, comfrey, or peppermint. More elaborate concoctions might use these or other ingredients in a poultice or in a lotion rubbed directly on the place that hurt. Hot or cold packs were also recommended. To modern headache sufferers, these solutions may seem quite reasonable, fairly familiar, and potentially comforting, but then as now, busy men and women with chores and duties to perform may not have had many opportunities to rest with a compress on their foreheads. (According to one advice book, for example, the victim of a nervous headache was supposed to reapply hot wet cloths every three minutes. One suspects that servants would have to be involved.)[11] Mary Chesnut tells us she stayed in her room all day with a bad headache, but she at least had friends, relatives, and indeed slaves to attend to the rest of the household.

If one of her slaves, however, had had the headache, the patient's experiences would have been rather different. After the war, a St. Louis doctor reported how an old southern gentleman had dealt with his field hands: "whenever a slave complained of a headache, [the planter] would run his penknife into the tip of his nose and the headache would be relieved."[12] Given such care, it is perhaps doubtful that a slave would have ever admitted to having a headache to his or her mistress, and not surprisingly, headaches seem to have been reported even less often than they were among whites.[13]

It was far better, of course, to avoid headaches altogether. Preventive measures included liberal use of charms and talismans, but there was practical advice as well. Perhaps if Jefferson had heeded the counsel an English contemporary had given to a young gardener, the future president would have been spared much distress. The gardener in question, whose headaches, like Jefferson's, were periodical and severe, was instructed to enjoy a moderate diet, imbibe but little alcohol, to wear his hair short (unless he wore a wig, in which case he should shave his head twice a week), never to bathe his body but only his head and neck each morning "with the coldest water he can procure," to wear nothing too tight, to wash his feet, wear warm stockings, "and at every approach of his headache . . . apply about six leeches to his temples and behind his ears." No drugs except aperients (mild cathartics) were ever to be taken.[14]

The ingestion of medications for a headache was not uncommon in domestic treatment, but topical compresses and lotions seem to have predominated. With the exception of the opiates, however (and again, it must be emphasized that narcotics were considered the last resort, not the first), few of the potions described in the lay literature would be recognized today as possessing analgesic properties, and in fact they were not used as such—at least, not directly. This is not so odd as it may at first appear. In early nineteenth-century domestic treatment, it seemed far-fetched to suppose that a substance taken into the stomach should do nothing but kill a pain in the head. Besides, nothing in the repertoire seemed to do this. Even the opiates did far more than just eliminate pain. The narcotics had a profound effect on the mind as well as on the body, which is one of the reasons they were not used indiscriminately for moderate discomfort. Much domestic medical thought appears instead to have been based on the premise that ill health was due to something "bad" accumulating in the body. More often than not, these bad things were the noxious entities that collected in the digestive system because of indiscretions of diet or because of what is today euphemistically termed irregularity. After all, the stomach and bowels were very frequently discombobulated in all sorts of disorders; cleaning out these organs would generally do no harm and would quite likely do a lot of good. It stood to reason that intestinal poisons could cause a headache (just consider the familiar consequences of excessive alcohol consumption), so getting rid of them expeditiously was both sensible and practical. If the toxins were eliminated, the headache would fade away. Thomas Jefferson expressed just such a view when, in his letter to his daughter about his June 1790 migraine, he wryly hoped that an anticipated expedition on George Washington's yacht would provoke a bout of seasickness that would "carry off the remains of my headach [sic]."[15] So it is not surprising that many home headache remedies were purges, vomits, or items such as bicarbonate of soda, which soothed or regulated the digestive system in some fashion. Diaphoretics (substances that induce perspiration) and sialogogues (that induce salivation) were also popular, sweating and spitting being more discreet ways of expelling unwanted elements. Noxious entities could also be distracted by using counter-irritation to draw the poisons from one part of the body to another. Hence General Grant's mustard footbath for his sick headache: instead of bothering his head, the toxins would be lured to his feet.

It is difficult, however, to identify any remedial substance, whether internal or external, that had special popularity. The ingredients in domestic recipes were mostly (although not exclusively) derived from local botanical sources, but of the hundreds of plant species whose roots, leaves, stems, bark, or berries were desiccated, infused, boiled, mashed, or macerated in the service of headache treatment, not one could be said to have found general employment. Indeed, if we counted up every item, recipe, or practice that over the centuries has been endorsed by someone, somewhere, as a headache remedy, the list would run to many pages. Whether any of them got rid of a headache, however, is another question altogether. From the modern perspective, it seems unlikely, but our definition of a headache cure is conditioned by events that we have yet to describe. In the nineteenth century, rapid relief from pain without the use of narcotics seems not to have been anticipated. The best anyone could reasonably expect was relief in a few hours. Compresses and bed rest did well enough under the circumstances.

Nonetheless, not all headaches were left to home care. Physicians, in fact, were often called on to deal with the very stubborn and puzzling cases that domestic medicine could not cope with, in addition to seeing countless more patients whose headaches were simply an aggravating accompaniment to their other ailments. And doctors were certainly aware of the myriad "ordinary" headaches that afflicted the population with "the utmost frequency," even if they were rarely asked to treat them.[16] Unlike folk healers, however, American doctors had a mature and well-established body of arcane medical knowledge, derived from more than two millennia of philosophy, theory, and investigation, upon which foundation they based their claims to professional status and authority (claims that, as we shall see, the public did not necessarily heed). Although not all who called themselves physicians had mastered this knowledge or were of one mind about its principles and practices, and although there were enough dissenting voices to create alternative medical systems and sects (such as homeopathy and hydropathy), most doctors in the nineteenth century were mainstream (that is, regular or orthodox) physicians who shared certain notions about health, disease, and treatment that stretched back to Galen and Hippocrates. They especially prided themselves on being "scientific," labeling all others as empirics—or worse.[17]

Generalizations about professional practitioners are nevertheless problematic: medical thinking changed more rapidly and drastically in the nineteenth century than in any previous hundred-year period. Divisions within regular medicine could be just as wide as those between sects, and doctors' education in the sciences they praised was often quite meager.[18] Even so, for most of the century, at the heart of virtually all accepted notions of health and illness was the view that "disease [was] essentially a systemic imbalance," "a condition of the individual man," a "dyscrasia" that upset the body's usual arrangement or constitution.[19] As a general principle, this holism held sway whether the constitution was thought of in terms of the classical humors or the more recent notions of tissue systems and cellular pathologies contributed by nineteenth-century science.

Put in its simplest terms, and without doing justice to the sophistication and complexities that these ideas often contained, a body was sick when it was out of balance with itself or its environment.[20] Restoring the balance restored health. A disease was therefore not a "thing" with an independent existence that invaded the body but was the body's response to a stimulus of some kind, the way a bruise is the body's response to a hammer blow. The bruise is real enough, but it cannot be said to exist apart from the unfortunate thumb. Diseases were likewise idiosyncratic reactions to diet, the weather, emotions, bad habits, new activities, and so forth; the degree and nature of the response were dictated by the individual's constitution. For orthodox physicians in the first two-thirds of the century, identifying what had become unbalanced in any particular patient and then determining what treatment would correct it were among the principal challenges of their profession and what (in their own minds, at least) gave them an advantage over domestic and sectarian healers who aimed their treatments at the obvious—at the symptoms themselves, mistaking them for the actual illness. Worse, some empirics thought diseases were entities that could be chased out of the body with specific cures, as if all patients were exactly the same and responded in the same way to a particular treatment.

Orthodox doctors, on the other hand, considered specific treatments (with a few important exceptions such as cinchona or quinine in intermittent fevers and mercury in syphilis) to be tantamount to quackery and instead understood symptoms to be important diagnostic clues that needed careful assessment before a course of treatment was undertaken. The intention was to foster a "constructive metamorphosis" of the whole system, not merely to patch up one part or another. Physicians thus had to be keen observers of facial expressions, complexion, movement, tone of voice, the pulse, and other signs; they also had to rely heavily on what the patients themselves told them—descriptions of nausea, chills, and other distresses, their customary habits, any unusual events in their lives, and their various aches and pains. The headache—that most common of pains—was accordingly a diagnostic clue of great importance.

Unfortunately, the very omnipresence of headaches also rendered them highly perplexing. The ancient Greek physician Galen (whose humoral system became the basis for most subsequent European medical concepts) had simply assumed that *any* humoral imbalance caused the excess to collect in the head. Eighteen hundred years later, physicians found themselves no further along, noting in some frustration that "there are instances of [headache] being occasioned by every thing that weakens the body."[21] The plethora and variety of headaches meant that ascertaining the causes of any particular one might prove very difficult indeed. Short sharp pain, ceaseless throbbing, prolonged dull aching, intermittent waves of intense pressure, perhaps nausea, perhaps not, frontal, occipital, temporal—the only thing headaches had in common was the misery they caused. In fact, it was their maddening diversity that ensured that headaches would always be construed as symptoms of other, more fundamental problems. Only the migraine, with its distinctive aura, sensitivity to light, and other features, came close to being considered a disease in itself, and even migraines were known to occur sometimes without pain; in these cases, too, the headache was but one manifestation of a more basic dysfunction. Consequently, the list of possible causes could be long and unwieldy. According to a medical textbook of the early nineteenth century (reflecting the fairly eclectic nature of medical thought at that time), headaches could be the result of factors that were internal (causes in the head), external (causes not in the head), idiopathic, sympathic, protopathic, deuteropathic, symptomatic (all specialized terms related to contemporary medical theory), sanguineous, bilious, phlegmatic (that is, humoral), febrile, inflammatory, rheumatic, catarrhal, arthritic, scorbutic, venereal, hypochondriacal, hysterical, or convulsive.[22]

One hundred years later, a diagnostic handbook with an even longer list named more than one hundred possible causes—but used a terminology that reflected some of the scientific developments that had occurred in the interval (trigeminal neuralgia, pharyngitis, cirrhosis of the kidney, dengue, chlorosis).[23] At one time or another in the nineteenth century, headaches were also ascribed to worms in the brain, irritation of the nerves or spasms of the blood vessels, too much blood or too little blood in the general circulation, in the brain, or in the scalp. They could be caused by head lice, high blood pressure, low blood pressure, eyestrain, bad food, unusual food, too much food, too little food, indigestion, fatigue, heat, cold, too much sun, too much hair, hats too tight, collars too tight, working too hard, thinking too much. A favorite cause, much resorted to, was constipation. And of course, thousands upon thousands were familiar with the headaches that occurred after drinking too much.[24]

Although some intrepid researchers tackled the subject from time to time, headaches on the whole did not receive as much scientific attention as other phenomena. Besides, their general lack of real danger and their transience ensured that practitioners did not wrestle with them overmuch. Yet they were not dismissed as irrelevant. Nor, despite the general recognition that more women than men complained of headaches, were they described as a "female complaint." (Menstrual causes were not emphasized. The preponderance of female victims was usually attributed to the greater sensitivity of women's bodies rather than to some specifically "female" element.) Doctors always understood that a headache could "[torment] its subjects by severe pain . . . [and] unfit them for the active duties of life."[25] Throughout the nineteenth century, orthodoxy considered pain of all kinds to be physically real, exaggerated by some patients, perhaps, but not created by the mind.[26] Even though emotions and intellectual activities such as deep thought were considered to be possible causes of head pain, the pain was as real as that caused by toxins or trauma, physically affecting some structure in the body—the blood vessels, for example, or even the brain itself.

Take Silas Weir Mitchell's description of a young headache victim, a sixteen-year-old boy, who, "while oppressed under certain family troubles, still contrived to lead his class at the high-school." Unfortunately, he began to get headaches so severe they prevented him from studying: "the slightest methodical use of the brain cost him hours of pain." However, "the pain was absent, or rare, as long as he rode horseback, or played ball, or idled at the seashore."[27] Mitchell, who later became famous for his rest cure for nervous disorders, seems to have accepted this at face value and did not even hint that the boy might be pretending to have headaches, or was conjuring them in some fashion, in order to avoid the stress of scholarship or of pleasing his family. Not only were these headaches as real as those caused by poisons or disease, but they appeared to Mitchell to be analogous to overuse of the muscles. And just as he believed patients who said their arms and legs ached from too much labor, he believed that this teenager's head ached from "undue cerebral taxation." If symptoms were to have any function at all in a discursive medical practice, doctors *had* to assume that their patients were telling the truth about them, at least most of the time. Hence they appraised reports of headaches (and pain in general) as seriously as reports of dizziness or double vision. Patients did not often face skeptics. They did, however, face doctors who did not necessarily endorse analgesia or pain control as the primary goal of treatment.

Instead, physicians focused on the pain's cause. Analgesics would only conceal the symptom, not cure the condition. Because pain usually indicated that something had gone wrong in the body, it was demonstrably foolish and harmful to mask it with drugs before its source had been determined. An often-cited paradigm was the toothache. The rotten tooth might continue to do damage even when the happily drugged patient could not feel it. The only cure was extraction. Clearly, eliminating the cause of the pain was superior to simply ameliorating it. With most kinds of pain, the part of the body that hurt was also the part that had something wrong with it, and the doctor could direct his attention appropriately, ascertaining the cause without much difficulty. Headaches, unfortunately, were not so obliging. More often than not, they seemed to indicate that something was amiss somewhere else in the body. For unknown reasons, an upset stomach, a fever, or a disease like syphilis could signal its presence by a pain in the head. Only a few cases could, like Mitchell's teenager, be ascribed to brain fatigue or other "capital" causes. The majority of causes were arcane, obscure, or ambiguous. There is no other disorder, said one of the few headache researchers of the period, "which more taxes the experience and scientific knowledge of the physician, or requires closer observation in elucidating its nature and removing its obscurity."[28] Said another practitioner: "There is scarcely any other complication, to which the human system is heir, which causes the patient more continued misery, and the physician more annoyance and disgust with his powers of diagnosis, and with the workings of his remedies, than headache."[29] This most common of symptoms, in other words, was most uncommonly problematic.

The easiest course of action, surely, would have been for physicians to prescribe a narcotic and hope for the best. Some doctors in fact complained that this was exactly what large numbers of their colleagues did. But in public, orthodox practitioners declared themselves to be above such empiricism. By explaining the patient's predicament in terms of arcane causes based on learned theories, doctors demonstrated the scientific underpinnings of orthodoxy and could therefore confidently determine the most suitable therapeutic response for a headache or any other ailment, which was usually expressed in a prescription of some kind. Fortunately, concepts of constitutional imbalance also supplied a rational guide for therapy: one could restore equilibrium by counteracting whatever was deficient or excessive. In the seventeenth and eighteenth centuries, this had evolved into a complex and sometimes baffling array of recipes that could involve dozens of ingredients. By the middle of the nineteenth century, a prescription rarely required more than a few items, but it could be a complicated undertaking nonetheless and was still considered to be representative of what made orthodoxy superior. Although they shared medical concepts with the general population, physicians believed they had a more complete understanding, deeper insights, greater wisdom. The prescription was evidence of this. Written in abbreviated Latin and ancient symbols, it also protected doctors' special knowledge from being too generally available to the public and was therefore an important symbol of their professional ideals.[30]

George Wood, professor of materia medica and therapeutics at the University of Pennsylvania, summarized the basic principles of orthodox prescribing as they were understood at midcentury.[31] Once the doctor had established the diagnosis, he had to weigh the available therapeutic approaches in light of the patient's idiosyncrasies and any peculiarities of the environment. He also had to keep several precepts in mind. Because blood in Western medical thinking retained its ancient position as the seat of many dyscrasias, *depletion* (a diminution of the blood) was a therapeutic principle of great value, even though by Wood's day it might not be achieved by bloodletting as often as formerly.[32] Cathartics, diaphoretics, emetics, and anything that promoted secretions were considered to accomplish the same ends.

In contrast to depletion, *repletion* required that the doctor increase the quantity of blood, most often by means of the patient's diet, by the use of tonics, or by stimulating the appetite. Indeed, *stimulation*, "the exaltation of any or all of the vital functions above the state in which they may happen to exist at the time when the stimulating measures are resorted to," and its opposite, *sedation*, were other important therapeutic principles for the

practitioner to keep in mind. Counter-irritation or *revulsion* diverted the
pathology from one seat in the body to another. Cathartics, said Wood, "act
very powerfully upon this principle in the relief of inflammation and congestion, though they may be employed chiefly in reference to their deplet-
ing power." Diversion was also accomplished by *supersession*, which
replaced one disease with another, a concept that explained why quinine
and arsenic were so successful in intermittent (that is, malarial) fevers:
these drugs "establish their own morbid impression, in the absence of the
[malarial] paroxysm; and the system, being thus occupied at the moment
when the disease was to return, is incapable of admitting it."[33]

Other authors elaborated additional points that had to be kept in
mind. Women and children tolerated harsh medicines less easily than did
men. The patient's race (including nationality) affected the prescription:
effeminate peoples were—like women—less able to bear up under aggressive treatment. Habits and lifestyles could alter the effect of medications,
as could the patient's mental state, religious beliefs, or indeed, belief in
the doctor.[34] Any factor at all could influence therapeutic choices and
might in some instances preclude the use of drugs altogether, leaving
treatment solely to diet or physical agents (such as cold water in fever). In
any event, these decisions required a full understanding of the patient's
own condition, needs, and wishes as well as the full exercise of the doctor's
own judgment, based on his knowledge, experience, and insight. It was
also not an undertaking for the timid or faint of heart.

Because many remedies for headaches were based on depletion, they
included a large proportion of emetics and cathartics. In this, professional
and domestic notions were similar. But physicians also tended to embrace
powerful mineral drugs such as calomel and antimony or to employ high
doses of botanics that domestic healers were not so willing to use. The
alkaloids, for example (powerful plant extracts such as quinine, morphine,
and strychnine, newly discovered in the early decades of the nineteenth
century), could be fatal in very small doses. Overall, the harsh and painful
attributes of doctors' drugs (and the debilitating effects of bloodletting,
which was also a professional monopoly) were the hallmarks of regular
medicine. To modern eyes these therapies appear spectacularly unpleasant (not to mention worthless) and hardly deserving of the term *heroic*,
which is often used to describe them (and which is more appropriate if

applied to the patients).[35] Although American doctors may not have been as guilty of these practices as some (then and now) have thought, and a significant number of physicians were in fact so skeptical of these treatments that they became virtual therapeutic nihilists, adopting an expectant or "wait and see" approach that relied on the healing power of nature, vigorous remedies vigorously applied remained the basis of most regular treatment until after the Civil War.

This style of practice was also what patients expected and even may have demanded. Fellow practitioners might have been impressed by a doctor's knowledge of theory and esoterica, but the public was impressed by what he actually *did*. It was "expected of the physician by common consent," as one practitioner noted, "to do something."[36] Activity was crucial because it "gave the physician his professional reputation."[37] Professional identity, in fact, depended on it.[38] Because the prescription represented the doctor's knowledge and competence, and was the chief means by which his expertise was conveyed to the patient, for any physician the art of prescribing was "a point intimately connected with his success as a practitioner."[39] For his patients, knowledgeable in the general concepts of therapeutic evacuation, that meant the prescription was expected to *produce an effect*. Simply feeling better was not proof at all of the doctor's skill. Headache sufferers therefore took their medications in anticipation of needing the chamber pot or the emesis basin close at hand. They were usually not disappointed. As a recalcitrant and stubborn phenomenon, headache found itself the target of some particularly energetic treatments.

By the early decades of the nineteenth century, prescriptions tended to be much simpler than they had been in earlier times, although complexity might be retained by having a series of recipes. In cases of sick headache, for example, a practitioner in 1822 first recommended a laxative (rhubarb or perhaps calomel) or an emetic (ipecac), followed by a mixture of prepared rust of iron, powdered columbo root (calumba, *Jateorrhiza palmata*, imported from Africa), and orange peel, to be taken twice a day for four weeks. Immediate pain relief does not appear to be the goal, and none of the ingredients was considered analgesic. The recipe instead focused on repairing the digestive system. (Calumba was a bitter stomach tonic, although in large doses it was an emetic and cathartic.) The rationale was the "sympathetic connection" between the stomach and the head—the former organ being responsible for the latter's distress rather than the other way around.[40] By far the majority of headache treatments prescribed in the nineteenth century reflected this point of view. It was a popular concept with a long life: as one journal noted in 1917, "there may be an occasional case of headache that does not need a cathartic," but in that case an enema could be given instead.[41] Even when headaches were thought to be caused by something not connected with the digestive system, a laxative would do the patient no harm.

When the nervous system was involved, headaches could be treated with various sedative preparations, including bromides, cannabis (especially useful in dealing with nausea), or bloodletting. Stimulants such as caffeine were also used—again, with the intention of targeting whatever was postulated as the underlying cause of the pain. Some fortunate patients were prescribed champagne; some less fortunate ones had jets of hot air forced into their noses and sinuses. Some even had blistering lotions applied to their shaved heads or leeches inserted in their nostrils. ("It is hardly necessary to add that, in the application of leeches to the septum, care should be taken to prevent the passage of the animals into the nasal cavity.")[42] When an underlying disease such as syphilis or malaria was identified as the root cause, mercurials or quinine, respectively, were ordered. Other causes such as bad teeth or eyestrain could be treated with tooth extraction or spectacles, and some hope of success.[43] But although there might be some successes, there always seemed to be an endless stream of patients whose headaches defied even the most confident physician. Few treatments were in any case expected to provide immediate relief. It sometimes took days or even weeks before the pain abated, despite daily visits from the doctor.[44] The temptation to resort to the opiates was strong, and many doctors no doubt succumbed. But their colleagues constantly warned them of the dangers: addiction, constipation, and a lethargy that "put the patient to bed thereby incapacitating him from business, which to some is a very serious matter."[45] Only on rare occasions were narcotics appropriate.

Not all professional advice was unpleasant, however. The best way to deal with headaches was to avoid getting them in the first place. Throughout the nineteenth century, most physicians advised their patients to avoid precipitating causes such as too much sun, rich food, wine, or over-work. This could be accomplished by establishing good habits of diet, drink, exercise, fresh air, and recreation appropriate to the constitution of each individual.[46] A number of American doctors lamented, however, that such good habits were foreign to their fellow countrymen, who had grown soft and weak under the influence of "the advanced state of civilization." Moreover, even as early as 1822, this luxuriant life was itself the cause of the "annual increase" in the number of headaches. An abstemious regimen was therefore necessary.[47] For those who could afford it, a change of scene or climate achieved the same goal far more agreeably: traveling for the sake of one's health was a fashionable, if expensive, therapy very popular with the leisured classes in all eras. But when prevention failed, the repertoire of pukes, purges, blisters, and lotions was waiting in the wings.

The unpleasantness of typical orthodox treatments had of course not gone unchallenged. Alternatives to regular medicine were becoming more conspicuous in American society by the mid-nineteenth century and included (besides home care and self-treatment) hydrotherapy, vegetarianism, homeopathy, Thomsonianism, botanical (or "Indian") doctoring, and later, Christian Science, among others. To some degree, these systems shared orthodoxy's view of illness as a disordered constitution but differed on how to restore balance and—in the opinion of the regulars—were seriously deficient in theory and science. Thomsonians, for example, saw cold as the culprit in all ailments and prescribed vegetable drugs thought to possess warming properties. Other botanic practitioners (later known as eclectics) favored a puke-and-purge regimen that differed from orthodoxy mostly in the use of less violent remedies, being especially hostile to mineral drugs like calomel.[48] Homeopathy, on the other hand, looked upon symptoms not as signs of dyscrasia but as the body's own attempts to heal itself. Guided by the doctrine that "like cures like," homeopaths used medicines that mimicked the symptoms of the disease but in such attenuated amounts that they were virtually absent from the prescription. If homeopathy did not cure, at least it did no harm. For that reason alone, this sect posed a particular challenge to the regulars because it was attractive to many Americans who were dissatisfied with more conventional medical systems. Yet homeopathy too was thwarted by the headache: "In no disease do we derive less help from pathology . . . ; in none are we so utterly dependent upon phenomena."[49] Its categories of headache types were therefore just as numerous as in regular medicine. One self-help book of 1889 described forty kinds: "*Pressive* headache, as if everything would come out at the forehead"; "*throbbing* in one or other temple; *drawing, tearing* headache"; "Pain like a *heavy weight at the top* of the head."[50] Each variety had its own remedy, but in the end, homeopaths were no more successful than regular doctors in solving the riddle of headache.

Thus, by about 1880, regular, alternative, and domestic medical practices appear to have arrived at more or less the same point with respect to headache treatment. Purges were among the most common remedies because they were an efficient method of ridding the body of what ailed it—a notion that could be accommodated by all medical philosophies (homeopathy excepted). Regular doctors, however, were more likely to also engage in lengthy and learned discourse about the nature of the underlying pathology. Moreover, their focus on causes and their understanding of contemporary medical theories allowed them to offer a greater variety of remedies (and a more confusing array of explanations) than most other practitioners, but unfortunately from the victim's point of view, such erudition was moot.[51] No one—unless willing to use opiates—expected or offered immediate relief from pain.[52] Moreover, regular doctors considered pain relief alone to be misguided, an empiric's response to a complicated, abstruse, and highly individual set of circumstances. Far better to identify and deal with pain's source. But to headache sufferers, pain *was* the problem. We know this not so much because they said so but because of their reaction to the arrival of the first nonnarcotic painkillers in the mid-1880s, as we shall see presently. Until those chemicals became available, however, Americans with headaches had to comfort themselves with other measures drawn from the vast repertoire of nature's resources and the human imagination. In this sense, their options were unlimited.

2

Drug Supply in
Nineteenth-Century America

Whether they had headaches or not, Americans loved to take medicines. "We swallow [them] as greedily as the catfish swallows the schoolboy's bait," noted a Tennessee doctor in 1852, commenting on a characteristic that ever since colonial times had supported a flourishing drug trade.[1] By the 1830s and 1840s, this trade had evolved into a variety of suppliers who between them could provide virtually any item that anyone in the country might want, no matter how exotic.[2] There were large wholesalers of indigenous and imported raw botanicals, and small local manufacturers (often attached to a pharmacy) of items such as quinine, strychnine, and morphine. These chemicals, known as alkaloids and derived from botanicals, were difficult or impractical to make outside a pharmacy laboratory but were finding considerable use in medical practice.[3] A growing number of firms produced tinctures (alcohol-based solutions) and fluid extracts as conveniences that saved the doctor or local apothecary a good deal of time and bother. In addition, there was a wide variety of specialty manufacturers, specialty importers, and companies making ready-to-use recipes (more about these later). Dealing in all these goods were the jobbers— local, regional, and national distributors—who combined the importation, reprocessing, and manufacturing of drugs with the production or sale of virtually anything that could be considered chemical or medicinal. Paints, rat poisons, bug killers, fabric dyes, hair dyes, varnishes, wood preservatives, wines, and whiskies joined opium, morphine, quinine, bloodroot, henbane, cohosh, and imported French soap in these companies' catalogs.

Despite the specialized and potentially dangerous nature of many of their wares, no drug supplier and virtually no state or federal laws in the nineteenth century required that customers have professional credentials or proof of medical expertise before drugs were shipped to them.[4] So long as Americans lived great distances from doctors or renounced orthodox medicine as just so much bunk, in the popular view they were entitled to doctor themselves.[5] So long as they had an appetite for drugs, they were entitled to buy them without hindrance. Drugs were natural items, found in the public domain, gifts from Providence like fire and other necessary but hazardous things. If customers poisoned themselves, the supplier was only at fault if he had supplied an incorrect or adulterated item.[6] Restricting access would have been seen as unjustifiable, contrary to common sense, and perhaps unpatriotic as well as unprofitable. Directly or indirectly, supply houses in the antebellum United States depended for much of their business on ordinary citizens and domestic practitioners, and therefore solicited customers from all walks of life. Any newspaper, especially those published in small towns, was replete with local druggists' advertisements that listed not only their own products but those from the large suppliers they dealt with. Harwood and Williams of Fayette, Mississippi, for example, announced that they bought their "Syrup of Iodide of Iron" from Schieffelin Company in New York, one of the biggest of the New York jobbers.[7] Furthermore, even regular physicians—who in general were not very supportive of practices that competed with the medical profession—were not opposed to such open access, given the conditions in the country at the time. Doctors could not be everywhere at once. Self-care was a reasonable alternative, within limits. Besides, in the antebellum era, the medical profession was far too weak and disorganized to do much about it.[8]

The George B. Carpenter Company of Philadelphia, a typical jobber, reflects the reality of this medical world. Its 1835 catalog contained a wide array not only of drugs and chemicals but also of surgical instruments, books, glassware, and apparatus. Sales were pitched not just to doctors and chemists but to the whole spectrum of the population. The company obligingly listed the drugs a country storekeeper should always have on hand. There were kits, earmarked for country doctors, containing appropriate quantities of essential drugs (with labels in Latin or English, for $90 to

$100), along with a saddlebag version (with square jars and bearskin cover, for $25 filled or $15 empty of the drugs). Carpenter also provided a line of family medicine chests. City dwellers were advised to purchase chest number 1, costing $20 to $30 and consisting of a small, attractive piece of furniture that contained an assortment of useful remedies: cream of tartar, castor oil, calomel, paregoric (camphorated tincture of opium), Epsom salts, blistering ointments, and ipecac, among other items. Also included were glass measures, scales, and Carpenter's own *Dispensatory*, a book that listed "the properties and doses of each article most approved in Domestic Medicines" plus "a concise Description of Diseases, with directions for the treatment of such as are unattended with serious consequences, shewing also the best immediate measures to be adopted in those disorders and accidents which are destructive to life, when the physician is not at hand, or until his assistance can be procured."[9] This same *Dispensatory* accompanied the other versions of the medicine chest, each grade containing the articles appropriate to domestic care farther and farther from the centers of population: country folk, back-country folk, ships at sea. (Companies and stores that did business in the South similarly promoted medicine chests for plantations and steamboat use.)[10] Carpenter's products and the advice that accompanied them appear to have been well within the orthodox medical camp, but although some manufacturers adhered to sectarian lines, jobbers on the whole were fairly catholic. A customer was a customer. Homeopathic, botanic, and mineral remedies mingled in their product lists.

Nevertheless, although sectarians are usually thought to be far more sympathetic to self-prescribing, heterodox practitioners did not necessarily endorse homemade remedies. In homeopathy, for example, the correct dose was the *least* amount necessary to do the job, resulting in such dilutions that skeptics could not distinguish them from plain water. But to homeopaths these dilutions were most emphatically not mere water, and the method of obtaining them by repeated attenuations was an important aspect of their system. Consequently, homeopathic remedies generally could not be reproduced by domestic care-givers and, like orthodox drugs, had to be purchased from reputable suppliers.[11] Similarly, Samuel Thomson thought it prudent (and profitable) to make sure that "Genuine Thomsonian Medicines," "warranted pure and free from adulteration," were available only from authorized depots (in theory). But Thomson and his disciples could not control everything that was done in his name, and by the 1830s the movement had divided acrimoniously into true Thomsonians and eclectics. Many of the botanic medicines that eclectics favored were derived from indigenous plants and were vigorous enough as cathartics to became popular even in regular practice. They were quickly added to the jobbers' catalogs, although some botanic dealers became large distributors in their own right.[12]

There were also several drugless medical alternatives that became fairly popular, but most antebellum Americans continued to equate medicine with medications and on the whole gave their business to sects that used drugs. Moreover, despite widespread misgivings about physicians as a species, they gravitated toward remedies endorsed by a "Doctor." Not all men and women could diagnose their own ills or could distinguish black henbane from black cohosh, so medical advice and information were often as marketable as the medicines themselves. A significant number of periodicals, pamphlets, guidebooks, and other publications emerged from across the medical spectrum in the first half of the century to tell Americans what ailed them and how to cure it—often with remedies the author or publisher just happened to have for sale.[13]

In 1843, for example, Dr. Jesse Spear of Boston, a "celebrated Indian doctor" who had created his own "celebrated Indian Medicines" (not an Indian, Spear was clearly in the botanic camp), began to advertise them in his own biweekly *Boston Guide to Health and Journal of Arts and Sciences*, available for one dollar per year. This was not simply an organ for self-promotion. His paper, he said, was "a very desirable [one] for every family, on account of the many valuable recipes for many important medicines, and other articles, besides much useful instruction" that it contained. In it, he promised to provide "a sure remedy for Whooping Cough" and information about how to prevent colds and fevers. Readers lucky enough to be in New England could call for advice, gratis, at his Boston office; others would have to avail themselves of his Balm of Life or Grand Restorative Cordial. Unlike his consultation services, these celebrated medicines were not offered free of charge, but those who doubted their efficacy would be supplied with testimonials from satisfied purchasers.[14] Similarly, the *Thomsonian Botanic Watchman* of Albany, New York (1834, whose masthead pictured an Edenic landscape, with the caption "The sun of science arising upon the flora of North America"), and a host of other botanic periodicals all drove home the horrors of calomel and lauded the virtues of vegetable drugs— which fortuitously were available from the publisher or his agent, preformulated for the convenience of purchasers. And for their protection, as well. "Beware enemies who sell adulterated medicines," warned William Floyd, editor of the *Botanic Investigator* of Vicksburg, who then invited readers to Floyd and Brothers, the only Horton Howard agent in that Mississippi town, where they could safely purchase such items as Toothache Bark, Cholera Syrup, and Vegetable Pills. (Dr. Howard was engaged in a controversy with Samuel Thomson, hence the potential for sabotage.)[15]

In that they targeted the public for the specific purpose of self-treatment and were reticent about what they actually contained, these balms, cordials, and restorers could be called patent medicines. Yet the botanic newspapers frequently printed recipes and treatment methods from which they could make no money at all, so it is difficult to describe all the remedies or their proprietors as humbugs and quacks. Motivated by idealism perhaps more than profits, many of these little drug-and-newspaper businesses seem to have been run by true believers in health reform, and taken together, their message and their merchandise no doubt reached a respectably large audience. Furthermore, their very existence is testimony not only to Americans' ongoing concern for their health but to the public's active involvement in what course of action to take, which system to adopt, modify, or reject, which recipe to try, whose claim of therapeutic knowledge to believe. And if professional or purchased wisdom failed, antebellum Americans were always free to fall back on their own imagination and judgment. The public was therefore not inclined to deny itself even dangerous, potent medicines such as morphine and strychnine. All possible options remained available. Anyone could buy any substance from anywhere in the world and use it—on himself, at any rate—in any way he chose. What laws existed to restrict the practice of medicine to licensed physicians were impossible to enforce. Other than the regular physicians, few in America protested this situation or found it troubling, least of all the jobbers and other suppliers who profited from it.

Surely, then, somewhere in this omnium-gatherum headache sufferers should have found a decent remedy. But as we have already noted, this does not seem to have been the case. The botanic magazines, for instance, hardly even mentioned the complaint. If headache was discussed at all, the recommended course of action was a laxative or perhaps a vegetarian diet. Benjamin Colby's *Guide to Health,* one of the most popular Thomsonian handbooks, contained only one headache recipe (a snuff of bayberry, bloodroot, and sassafras bark) and did not include headache in its list of common medical problems and their treatments. Opium—a plant drug held in such high esteem by the regulars—was not revered in botanic circles for any illness.[16] It would never have been recommended for a headache. And homeopaths believed that analgesia would not only mask the clues to the underlying cause but would disturb the healing process itself.[17] In fact, the sects may have been less sympathetic to the problem than regular medicine was. Many sectarians had a puritanical streak and subscribed to the notion that high living, too much rich food and drink, or too many late nights was the source of much ill health; headaches were a good example of chickens coming home to roost. The ailment required moral reform rather than medical treatment. Besides, pain was man's lot in this world. It said so in the Bible.

But pain as a general problem was not altogether ignored in the nineteenth century. An increasingly secular society was becoming far less inclined to accept the providential nature of any type of suffering.[18] The introduction of surgical anesthesia in the 1840s was a dramatic example of this outlook, but the antislavery movement, women's movements, children's movements, societies for the prevention of cruelty to animals, and other humanitarian causes were also part of this antebellum trend; all were united by "a preoccupation with pain."[19] So when a Massachusetts shoemaker introduced a brew he called Painkiller to his fellow countrymen in the 1840s, he found many eager customers. He also introduced a new word to the language, and perhaps a new concept to medicine.[20]

Perry Davis was apparently not made of the stoic, uncomplaining stuff of his New England ancestors and did not suffer his numerous chronic and painful afflictions gladly. Desperate for relief, fed up with doctors of all stripes, and dissatisfied with existing remedies, he tried concocting his own. Around 1840 he came up with a recipe that worked. It worked so well that he felt it uncharitable to keep it to himself, so in 1845 he offered Perry

Davis' Painkiller to the rest of the world. Although several preparations available in the 1830s had included pain in their lists of curable conditions, Davis's invention was the first to identify itself primarily as an analgesic, with a word he made up himself. It "enjoyed almost instantaneous, worldwide success" and spawned a host of imitations.[21] Clearly, Davis had hit a nerve, so to speak. But he was neither a philanthropist nor a medical reformer. He belonged to no sect, apparently, except that of entrepreneur. His Painkiller was not a gift to suffering humanity. The word was registered as part of a trade name; the recipe he kept secret. Mr. Davis's invention, in fact, and the Pain Annihilators, Pain Extractors, and Pain Eliminators that followed in its wake were prime examples of patent medicines.

Patent medicines (also known as nostrums or proprietaries) originated in Europe in the seventeenth and eighteenth centuries as mass-produced and mass-advertised versions of common but complex prescriptions or of the special recipes of famous practitioners: Reverend Thomas Daffy's purgative Elixir, Dr. Patrick Anderson's cathartic Pills, Dr. Thomas Bateman's cough Drops were but three of the dozens that became popular.[22] Transported to the New World by the colonists, they served the needs of Americans who were not adept at practicing domestic medicine or who were unable or unwilling to consult a physician, yet who were just as eager as any other patriotic citizen to swallow drugs. Even the most ardent critic of medical bombast was likely to demand tonics and bracers or consider cathartics as part of the natural order of things. Patent medicines filled this need. Not entirely respectable because they appeared to prostitute medical wisdom for personal gain (and some were known to be utter frauds), many early patent medicines were nonetheless fashionable even with the medical profession, and no American drug wholesaler of the colonial and early republican period would be without a wide assortment. Until the early decades of the nineteenth century, these were largely venerable English brands, but by the time Perry Davis' Painkiller appeared, homegrown nostrums of all kinds had already started to proliferate. Indeed, they were becoming a veritable flood. These too were stocked by respectable drug suppliers and were sometimes used by respectable physicians, but their target market was the public, and many of them wooed that market by showing evident disdain for professional—especially orthodox—medicine.

By focusing on the public and developing strategies that appealed to

ordinary men and women, the nostrum makers became a distinct and independent branch of the American drug industry, growing less respectable
and more conspicuous over the decades, especially after the Civil War. In
1859 the output of the industry was fairly modest ($3.5 million according to
the census figures), yet one observer estimated that by 1883, annual sales
had already reached $40 million.[23] In 1900, the United States government
claimed that annual sales of patent remedies were nearly $59 million.[24]
Even after taking the increase in the population into account (from 31.5
million in 1860 to 75.9 in 1900), the per capita expenditure on patent
medicines soared in that forty-year period from eleven cents to
seventy-eight cents. Clearly the nostrum purveyors were on to something.
Promoted in the newspapers, the religious press, on billboards, barns, cliff
faces, and posters all over the country, endorsed by respectable persons
including members of the clergy and genteel society matrons, the miracle
potions and panaceas found a willing market. Some claimed to be the medicines that doctors themselves depended on; others claimed to eliminate
the need for doctors altogether. As early as 1841, one medical publication
complained: "The newspapers are crowded with advertisements of nostrums and certificates of cures, physicians and medical science are grossly
caricatured and reviled; pills are beginning to form an important item of
domestic manufacture, and elixirs are sold for their weight in gold."[25]

James Harvey Young's pioneering studies of the nostrum business in
the United States are still the most thorough and entertaining accounts,
although he begins with the premise that all the items in question were
dangerous, ridiculous, or useless and their promoters either frauds or
fools.[26] Not all nostrums can be painted with the same brush, however, and
their success was not simply the result of the chicanery of their makers.
More sympathetic historians have noted that the same desire for medical
reform that motivated sectarian practitioners also motivated some patent
medicine makers.[27] (As mentioned earlier, many botanic recipes seem to
fall into this category.) The success of the nostrums in general, however,
can be attributed to the fact that they were widely and lavishly advertised
in an era in which no regulations restricted what the recipe contained or
what claims could be made about it.[28]

With so many products in competition, all claiming to be unique, potent, and free from harmful ingredients, each patent medicine maker had to find something that distinguished his goods from those of his rivals. Early newspaper advertising had usually been fairly prolix and unimaginative, constrained by contemporary printing technology to words rather than images. The first numbers of the *New York Illustrated News* in 1859, for instance, carried patent medicine publicity that consisted almost entirely of text with modest headline type, not entirely distinguishable from the news columns. Yet by 1862, illustrations accompanied many drug (and other) advertisements; the size and font of both text and headlines were varied. The advertising in general had become very noticeable. In this particular case, of course, the fact that the *News* was an illustrated paper may have accelerated the transition, but other publications from this era also began to carry much more "artistic" ad copy, with nostrums leading the way.[29]

Nostrum makers rapidly developed a style of presentation that drew to some extent on the fanciful imagery and visual attractions of the traveling medicine shows that had evolved in the colonial and early republican periods, and that connected products with specific images of vigor, beauty, youth, and wholesomeness as well as mystery and arcana.[30] Thus distinctive trademarks, especially those incorporating cabalistic signs, Indians, and mythological creatures, became important marketing tools. A few nostrums that targeted particular segments of the market, such as the soothing syrups for babies and treatments for female disorders, developed imagery appropriate to those customers, but most nostrums had universal markets in mind and therefore adopted trademarks and symbols with wide appeal.[31] Elaborate labels with imaginary or exotic landscapes, depicting the triumph of glowing health over the suffering wrought by disease, all helped convey the notion that without the product in question, the individual would be a miserable, decrepit wretch.

Other strategies were also attempted in the effort to find an advantage in this competitive market. Nostrums were apparently among the first consumer goods packaged at the factory in household sizes, ensuring that the purchase did not go home nameless, wrapped in anonymous brown paper. Package inserts, trade cards, or other material that had some further function as calendars or decorations were also a common feature.

Some firms even patented the shape of their bottles.[32] The name of the product, too, was obviously important, but until fairly late in the nineteenth century most nostrums went under the monikers of their inventors—Brandreth's Pills, Hostetter's Bitters, Hood's Sarsaparilla. John Hamlin added a term and sold Hamlin's Wizard Oil for decades, and several vendors adopted Indian names.[33] Later, Pink Pills for Pale People, Pe-ru-na, Castoria, and others gained fame. Underlying all these remedies, however, was the implicit or explicit guarantee of a cure. A nostrum that was understated in its claims could not survive for long.

Competition was fierce. Consequently, nostrum manufacturers did not find common cause until 1881, when a number of the best-known companies formed the Proprietary Association of America (PAA) to lobby Washington to remove the lingering Civil War tax on alcohol and similar "burdens that may oppress the trade." The organization went on to foster the other interests of its growing membership by using their power as advertisers.[34] The PAA became notorious for threatening to pull its members' advertising from newspapers whose editors supported any legislation, state or national, that the nostrum industry did not like.[35] Patent medicine makers were particularly averse to suggestions such as one made by a member of the Michigan State Medical Society in 1885, advocating a label law that would require a disclosure of contents, but this proposal, like more than a hundred other food and drug bills introduced into Congress after the Civil War, went nowhere, allegedly because of the drug lobby.[36]

The PAA did not want to be seen as merely mercenary, however, and was alert to the impact of science on contemporary medicine as well as to Americans' growing concerns for their health in the post–Civil War era. The association therefore always maintained that its members' products were placed "on the solid foundation of medical success," pointing out that the nostrums they sold had in fact emanated "from the intellect of many of the best members of the medical fraternity." Besides, their products were at least as safe as the concoctions doctors themselves prescribed.[37] Anyone doubting that fact need only read the *Boston Globe* for Monday, 17 August 1885. A good portion of the front page and the entire second page were devoted to endorsing the patent medicine industry and its products, reminding readers in no uncertain terms that nostrums had stood the test of time, were familiar, trusted, and "simply afford[ed] a known remedy for a known ailment." Moreover, no one was forced to buy them.[38]

In addition to newspaper editors, the PAA also had a close relationship with a number of legislators, both at the state and federal levels. The PAA's own records are not specific but suggest the organization had a certain amount of "influence" in the political arena. In 1884, for example, legislation had been proposed that would require all proprietaries be endorsed by Congress before being advertised through the mail. Concerned, the PAA drafted a letter that "was placed by trusty and influential persons in the hands of the Committee of the House of Representatives before whom the bill came, and the effect of the measure was such that the bill was not even reported by the Committee."[39] Saved from the burden (not to mention the embarrassment) of revealing trade secrets, the nostrum business proceeded as before, claiming to cure all known ailments with a minimum of inconvenience, for about a dollar a bottle.

Even at the end of the century, when one might suppose that the public had become somewhat more sophisticated and critical, the hyperbole with which patent medicines were advertised is astonishing. In the 1890s, for example, Radway's Ready Relief distributed a booklet announcing that the product possessed an "almost supernatural power" to cure and prevent cholera, typhoid, "and the most terrible plagues, pestilences, and deadly diseases known to the world." Griffith's Menthol Liniment "cures, *cures* mind you, coughs, colds, croup, whooping cough, sore throat, bronchitis, chills, cramps, pneumonia, etc.," when taken internally. Externally it dispatched lumbago, sciatica, lame back, headache (not entirely neglected, after all), bruises, sprains, and a host of other ailments. Readers of this heartening information found it in a little pamphlet interspersed with hints on proper etiquette and polite behavior—a good reason to keep the document for household reference. Paine's Celery Compound pitied its Canadian customers' lack of familiarity with the appearances of famous persons and so produced a little "album" containing portraits and brief biographies of Queen Victoria, the governor general, and a few other eminent individuals. The rest of the publication consisted of portraits of less famous but no less important men and women who bespoke the wonders of the medicine that had saved them from an early grave. All testimonials were warranted as genuine by a notary public.[40]

Because a nostrum was by definition a secret mixture and its manufacturer could at any time change its constituents or their proportions, it is not always certain what these concoctions actually contained. Analyses made at the turn of the century do not necessarily prove what the product might have consisted of fifty or even ten years earlier. It is evident, however, that before about 1860, most of the nostrums—even those that were marketed as safe alternatives to the unpleasantness of regular medicine—were either tonics (that is, basically anything with a bitter taste) or cathartics (any number of available drugs could produce this effect). In other words, although the individual may have employed the nostrum to combat a specific symptom or disease and was in fact encouraged to do so (in contrast to professional medicine's condemnation of specifics as quackery), a nostrum's effectiveness was not necessarily judged by its success at eliminating either the disease or the symptom but by the level of response it provoked, especially if it was a cathartic or emetic.[41] Just as in orthodox practice, the drug had to produce an effect in order to prove that purchasers were getting their money's worth.

So broad were the services performed by any of these concoctions that some commentators have suggested that patent medicine makers were the first merchants to recognize that they were not filling a need so much as creating one. It has been argued, for example, that in order to sell drugs to members of the public, manufacturers "first had to sell them a sense of themselves as diseased."[42] This view seems to be more valid when applied to the early twentieth century's onslaught on halitosis, acne, body odor, and other cosmetic problems. In the nineteenth century it is not likely that Americans needed advertising copy to tell them they were subject to fevers, consumption, dyspepsia, or rheumatism or that a neglected head cold might become pneumonia or worse. Their own medical traditions taught them that minor ailments could always become major ones. Although it is possible that in order to generate sales, medicine vendors took advantage of the population's fears by inventing or exaggerating dangers (impotence cures might be guilty of this), in the case of pain remedies, at least, they appear to be responding to a need already expressed.[43] Perry Davis did not have to look too far to find customers for his Painkiller.

The success of Perry Davis and his imitators is compelling evidence that midcentury Americans were indeed no longer willing to put up with pain. If the treatment they were prescribed by their doctors, whether regular or sectarian, did not give them the comfort they desired, patients turned to proprietaries. The manufacturers of painkillers embraced human frailties (indeed, they could scarcely exist without them), understood the public's desire for quick relief—and were there on the spot with the goods and the guarantees. Even the makers of the innumerable concoctions that merely included pain as just one of the things they could cure (in addition to dropsy, fevers, and warts) recognized that pain relief was a promise they should make. It is questionable, however, whether the remedies being offered might actually have been effective as painkillers.

It is commonly assumed that the chief appeal of nostrums in the nineteenth century was the large quantity of narcotics and alcohol they contained and that they in fact intoxicated consumers,[44] but it is not entirely clear just how widespread these substances actually were in patent medicines. Alcohol was certainly present in a large number of liquid preparations: even the vegetable compound of the famously teetotaling Lydia Pinkham was shown to consist of 18 percent spirits.[45] But it would be hard to get drunk on her concoction. Crammed with bitter herbs and other foul-tasting ingredients, it met the litmus test of medicinal products. It tasted awful, therefore it must be good. Besides, it was only intended to be taken by the spoonful, and it would take considerable resolve to swallow any more. Opiates, too, were camouflaged in disagreeable mixtures, but here the quantities that were claimed for them are much harder to document. Of about twenty-five hundred recipes published in 1899, only 5 percent or so contained any opium, morphine, codeine, cocaine, or cannabis. Moreover, a significant portion of these were ointments or other external remedies.[46] It is of course possible that earlier in the century more patent medicines did contain narcotics, and several categories—such as the infamous baby pacifiers—were notorious even in their own day for outrageous drugging, leading not just to narcotized infants but to "the early resort of our youth to tobacco and alcoholic stimulants."[47] Nevertheless, in an 1881 analysis of eight "painkillers" (the trade names were not provided), it was shown that six contained camphor, one had chloroform, some had ammonia, or red pepper, guaiac, myrrh, turpentine, or oil of sassafras; all contained alcohol, but not one contained a narcotic.[48] Had this list included Perry Davis' Painkiller, the analysts would indeed have found opium, along with a few other interesting ingredients (such as alkanet, an exotic herb thought to have sedative properties but that was also used as a red dye).[49] Undoubtedly there were many other "pain extractors" that contained opium or morphine: a list of more than thirty opiate-containing nostrums published in 1909 confirms that access to narcotics was never difficult in this period.[50] But the number of nostrums with narcotics appears to have been smaller than we might expect, even though there were absolutely no legal (and few moral) restrictions on their use until the second decade of the twentieth century.

At the same time, per capita consumption of the opiates was higher in the United States in the nineteenth century than in any other "civilized" country, with imports of opium soaring from 71,839 pounds in 1859 to an estimated 372,000 pounds in 1880. Observers were concerned: "Why so much larger quantity is consumed in this country than in Europe it would be difficult to determine. The greater number of persons suffering here with neuralgic troubles cannot possibly account for it."[51] Opiates are also powerful antidiarrheals and cough suppressants, and not all the imports would have been intended for painkilling, but the growing fear of addiction to narcotics (especially to morphine) after the Civil War created another alarming possibility.[52] Whatever the reasons, opiate imports kept increasing, reaching 587,121 pounds by 1892.[53] Sectarians blamed the orthodox doctors, regular practitioners blamed the patent medicine makers, the nostrum industry swore it did not use more morphine than anyone else, and social critics blamed the whole country, lamenting that Americans were losing their toughness.[54]

It is now generally acknowledged that the morphine habit was in fact created by regular doctors, in part because of their reliance on hypodermic injections to alleviate the distressing conditions of a particular class of patients. The typical drug fiend of the late nineteenth century, in fact, was a middle-aged,. middle-class white woman.[55] And although doctors were not inclined to use analgesics in headache or other minor pains, in cases of extreme need they were not reluctant to prescribe opiates, especially for its sedative properties. (Morpheus, god of dreams, was the son of Sleep, after all.) But the consumption of opium, whether professionally or self-prescribed or in nostrums, suggests at the very least that nineteenth-century Americans had a profound aversion to pain and were seeking ways to alleviate it. By identifying and focusing on this need, patent medicine companies never lacked for customers, and some of the vast quantities of opiates imported every year most certainly found their way into the nostrum factories.[56]

For many painful ailments it is likely that either prescribed or proprietary narcotics worked well enough. And perhaps the high alcohol content of nostrums may have provided a comforting sensation to those patients able to bear the taste long enough to consume a sufficient amount. But it is not at all clear whether the painkillers available up to the mid-1880s were found satisfactory by the vast majority of headache sufferers. Alcohol can exacerbate a headache, even in small amounts. Opiates could handle a severe headache fairly effectively, but at a price: putting the patient to sleep, rendering him too lethargic to continue with the day's activities, or making him an addict. As for the other ingredients that could be found in painkilling nostrums, these either were sedatives (e.g., camphor) or were employed for properties other than analgesic. In other words, it is uncertain whether headache victims would have found anything useful in the nostrum camp. The nostrums themselves seem to have recognized their limitations. A headache was never the first pain a painkiller could kill, appearing on most labels somewhere near the bottom of the list.

So despite the fact that for most of the nineteenth century headache sufferers had a variety of medical systems to consider, several kinds of practitioners to consult, and every medicine under the sun to purchase if they chose, no remedy seems to have achieved any particular popularity, all medical sects seemed equally helpless, and even the nostrum makers—who could cure cancer, consumption, and impotence in short order—did not offer much help. Headache remained the unpleasant experience it had always been, to be endured until it went away on its own or until the desperate victim took laudanum. Self-treatment, in other words, was certainly no worse than professional care. Yet in this same period, orthodox medicine both in America and abroad was beginning to make considerable progress, as new discoveries began to provide physicians with concepts in pathology and therapeutics that had the potential to revolutionize medical thought, professional practice, and the nation's health. By the second half of the nineteenth century, newspapers were acquainting American readers with the accomplishments of Pasteur, Lister, Koch, and others—accomplishments with which regular doctors claimed kinship, and that vindicated their avowed faith in science and theory. Eventually, both headache and headache remedies were to benefit from this progress. In the meantime, however, in the democratic medical environment of self-reliant patients and free choice, American doctors were a long way from the ideal, scientific practitioners that they aspired to be. Before they could convince the public that they were scientific professionals, they would have to convince themselves.

3

Doctors and the Drug Trade

Although many Americans in the nineteenth century were of the opinion that "approximately all doctors were parasites of society" and that at least two-thirds of them were going to hell, individual practitioners might be appreciated (however grudgingly) simply for being available, regardless of whether they were thought to be any good. Iowa farm boy Arthur Hertzler, who later became a doctor himself, reminisced about one country physician whose office contained "an old couch, three chairs, [and] a small table on which lay a great variety of inexpressibly dirty instruments" but who also "had the reputation of being a very fine doctor if one could find him sober." The trouble was that like many of his colleagues, he had a fondness for whiskey and, according to Hertzler, was under its influence most of the time. But unlike most of his colleagues, this practitioner had also been to medical school (two terms at Keokuk Medical College, one of the seventy or so proprietary schools in existence by the 1870s) and had more books in his office ("five big ones and three little ones") than young Hertzler had ever seen in one place before. Although Hertzler did not recall any evidence that this man had even saved a life, much less done anything truly noteworthy, he nevertheless thought "there was something heroic about him" because he "lived for his patients" and ignored his own comfort to sit with a sick child or do battle with mud and snow whenever a call for help came from an outlying farm. (The whiskey simply fortified him.) What he lacked in medical refinement he made up for with the "spirit of service." Children and old ladies loved him, and when he died of pneumonia after his team dumped him (drunk) into the creek one night, patients who had never paid their bills when the doctor was alive helped pay for his funeral.[1] Such scenes must have been played out in many parts of the country, where, all griping aside, communities did not usually reject even self-taught or tipsy practitioners. These men had their uses and perhaps were better than nothing.

But not as far as everyone was concerned. Some of the most zealous critics of regular practitioners were neither sectarians nor outraged members of the public but other regular practitioners who thought there were far too many men like this Iowan who claimed to be doctors on the slimmest of credentials, who may have had humanitarian impulses but were more likely to be charlatans and quacks, and whose incompetence and ignorance tarred all physicians with the same brush. Ever since colonial times, the best-educated and most ambitious physicians had fought to create an autonomous, learned profession on the European model, but they had been stymied by the conditions and attitudes in the new world. State and local medical societies and academies had virtually no effect on medical practice. Laws that stipulated who qualified as a doctor differed widely from state to state and could not be enforced anyway; virtually anyone could hang out a shingle with "doctor" on it and get away with it. By midcentury, with new discoveries from Europe shaking the very foundations of medical thought, with exotic drugs becoming newly available as France and England expanded their empires into Asia and Africa, it was time to address the medical free-for-all in the United States more directly.

In 1847 a group of reform-minded, mostly East Coast practitioners formed the American Medical Association (AMA), the first national voice for regular physicians. Although it was to be many years before the AMA became a powerful and authoritative organization, its eventual success and its persistent championing of professional standards, ethical behavior, and scientific methods allow us to consider it the medium through which we can learn what the elites of regular medicine were thinking. We might therefore expect that because it was created "primarily to raise and standardize the requirements for medical degrees," the AMA would be particularly concerned with improving and rationalizing medical education, especially in therapeutics. But the AMA was and remained far too weak and disorganized to have much impact at this time. Distracted, too, by questions of fee splitting, doctors' incomes, and especially the relationship of regulars to sectarians (which was to be no relationship at all: members were forbidden to consult with irregulars), the AMA did not focus on education again until the turn of the century. This meant that for most of the 1800s, regular doctors diagnosed and prescribed with only a modicum of training, formal or otherwise, and even the best schools taught about drugs not in terms of pharmacological or therapeutic principles but "as a kind of cataloguing process."[2] Prescribing was an exhibition of memory, not of knowledge.

One freshman practitioner described what must have been a common scenario. Soon after graduating from an unnamed medical school in 1870, he faced a child with hives. Uncertain about what to do, the young doctor hesitated until the child's nurse suggested "Saleratus water." "Fortunately remembering that 'Sodae et Potassae Tartras' was the pharmacopoeial name of the salt I assumed all the dignity of a professor of Materia Medica and wrote a prescription for a weak solution which I felt certain could do no possible harm. The child recovered."[3] When it came to determining treatment, all physicians relied on personal judgment guided by experience. If they lacked either, they faked it. Eventually, like the Canadian James Langstaff (who practiced north of Toronto from 1849 until his death forty years later), they developed a confident array of favorite remedies that may or may not have reflected the therapeutics they learned in medical school but that certainly reinforced the notion that drugs and plenty of them were essential for any regular practitioner's success, and that in Langstaff's case included a considerable number of the harsh and unpleasant medicines for which regular doctors received so much criticism.[4] He favored tartar emetic, for example—a noxious antimony and potassium preparation—whose therapeutic and toxic effects were virtually indistinguishable.

Having spent about two years at Guy's Hospital in London, in addition to training at a proprietary school, Langstaff was actually better educated than many of his colleagues. He subscribed to some important journals and modified his therapeutics over the course of his career, but even so, his patients must have had a rough time of it. How much worse might it be for the patients of doctors with even less training? How well did doctors actually know how to use all the drugs at their disposal, especially after the

Civil War, when the foundations of medicine were changing so rapidly? For reformers and others interested in improving both the skills and the status of American practitioners, these were not idle questions. In trying to answer them, however, they also began to direct their attention to drug suppliers, without whom the doctors' activities would have been much abbreviated.

All the drugs that made their way from doctors to patients ultimately came from one of the wholesalers, jobbers, specialty manufacturers, or nostrum firms discussed in the previous chapter. As we noted, in the first half of the nineteenth century most of these companies looked upon the entire population of the United States as their potential market and made little distinction between professional and lay clients. Yet by about 1850, influenced by the new medical sciences and the increasing activities of medical reformers, as well as the embarrassing excesses of the nostrum trade, a small number of drug firms began to emphasize their scientific and professional characteristics. They were joined after the Civil War by several more firms, many of whose founders were pharmacists or doctors.[5] These manufacturers highlighted their commitment to the healing arts at the expense (or so they implied) of large profits.[6] Although the firms never formed a specific organization or swore an oath, their advertising and other literature reveal the attitudes they embraced. First and foremost, these firms rejected patents. A patent was a monopoly that might tempt a drug maker to charge a high price for potentially life-saving items, and no right-thinking manufacturer would hold the public hostage to this form of greed. Second, the companies avoided trade names for their products because these obscured the identity of the ingredients. Instead, the companies used only the nomenclature of the *United States Pharmacopoeia* (*USP*). Third, they identified all the constituents of any mixtures they sold and did not tolerate secret ingredients. But it was for their refusal to advertise directly to the public that these companies earned the designation "ethical," a term that came into general use some time after the Civil War.[7] By limiting their business to professional customers, these drug suppliers presented themselves as partners in reform. They shared regular medicine's opinion that self-medication should not be encouraged. They supported efforts to establish industrywide standards. They applauded physicians' claims to be the proper guardians of medical knowledge and conceded that it was the business of doctors—not drug makers—to make therapeutic decisions.

Because proper physicians were expected to prescribe from scratch using *USP* standards, an ethical company was not supposed to manufacture "finished" items such as pills, capsules, or preformulated mixtures. It could, however, offer products that were expensive, difficult, or tiresome to make—such as the alkaloids, which began to be mass manufactured almost immediately after their discovery. As it turned out, far from discrediting medical practice, many of these "manufactured" articles could enhance it. Alkaloids such as strychnine and atropine are highly poisonous even in very small amounts. Indeed, the galenical preparations of these drugs had always been dangerous, but the margin for error was more forgiving than with the alkaloids. An infusion of cinchona bark, for instance, could be drunk in two-ounce doses, but quinine had to be taken in grains. One grain of the botanical extract of nux vomica was a fatal dose for a large dog, but only one-eighth grain of strychnine was required for the same result.[8] Factory-made drugs were also (in theory) standardized to some extent, with manufacturers using the *USP* as the touchstone, which eliminated the uncertainties of medicines made directly from botanicals with unknown concentrations of active ingredients.[9] "It would be difficult for those who have not practiced medicine," said an anonymous author at midcentury, praising the new drugs, "to comprehend how much a conscientious physician suffers, in consequence of uncertain action of the preparations which he is compelled to dispense."[10] In using these manufactured preparations, the doctor could exhibit his therapeutic finesse, and these items quickly became acceptable even to the elite in the profession. As long as the factory product was just another ingredient in a prescription, it was simply a resource like any other, to be managed as the physician saw fit.[11]

Ethical firms were also not expected to engage in research. "Theoretical disquisitions and philosophical experimentation" were the prerogatives of practitioners and academics, although a company was free to adapt or alter an existing commodity in order to improve it in some way. Parke, Davis and Company of Detroit was unusual in that it actively sought new botanical remedies, even sending expeditions to remote parts of the country. It also encouraged American doctors to be more systematic in testing new medicines and described how a new drug ought to come into practice—a slow process that would take years of use under different conditions, with different kinds of patients closely observed ("but avoid all unnecessary staring").[12] Yet its own novelties were in fact very conventional medicaments (cathartics, tonics, and so forth), and ultimately individual practitioners were left to themselves to determine how well any of them worked: "Experience in the use of a remedy is the only reliable test of its merit."[13] It was only on the consensus of practitioners that the legitimacy of medicinal substances could be established. The ideal pharmaceutical company merely facilitated the introduction of these agents to the profession at large. If the item proved popular, all other firms quickly had it in stock. A monopoly, of course, would have been unethical. A firm created its clientele by being the first or the best or the cheapest—but not the only—supplier.

This ethical posture created a difficulty for the industry, however. Manufacturers were, after all, in business to make money. Yet for most of the century the major ethical companies carried virtually the same wares, a striking "overlap in product lines," all claiming the same standards of purity and excellence.[14] Unless the prescription specified the manufacturer (in which case the pharmacist was obligated to dispense that product), it was largely up to the druggist to decide which maker's item to use.[15] Quinine from one reliable supplier was very much like quinine from another reliable supplier. But if a company could somehow persuade physicians to prescribe *its* products, they would have a considerable advantage over their competitors. Thus, throughout the second half of the nineteenth century, the marketing strategies of most ethical drug firms were attempts to entice doctors to prescribe a particular make of medicine while not appearing to violate professional principles. The various means they employed to sell as much of their wares as they could stood in contrast to the noble prose with which they described themselves and their products. Their commercial activities certainly belie the notion that "old-time drug companies were limited to a small amount of restrained advertising in professional journals and occasional visits to physicians by company sales representatives, stressing the quality of the company's product line."[16] Quite the contrary: many of the marketing strategies and advertising techniques that are serious points of dispute among industry, physicians, government agencies, and consumers today originated and flourished more than a century ago.[17]

Early nineteenth-century physicians rarely commented on how they found out about new products. Occasionally, a doctor's memoir might note that he had been impressed by pharmaceutical innovations in his youth, without saying how he had learned of them.[18] Somehow, items associated with a particular firm became well known, as evidently happened with the Philadelphia concern of Brown and Rosengarten. Their morphine became so popular that "Mr. Rosengarten . . . estimated his production of it during the first three years [to about 1830] at 5,000 ounces a year," but we can only speculate on how this popularity was achieved—hand bills, word of mouth, free samples, or just good press, such as the article in the *American Journal of Pharmacy* in which this statistic appeared.[19]

By the last decades of the century it is clear that many companies were energetically courting potential clients. One young doctor wrote home in May 1900 about a visit to the Parke-Davis facilities in Detroit, where he and his fellow medical students were "entertained at a glorious banquet where we sat at table for three hours," and where no doubt the conversation included more than one reference to the company's products. (Whether the letter writer became a convert to them we never find out.)[20] The therapeutic skeptic William Osler once mentioned the irritating prevalence of the traveling salesman, the " 'drummer' of the drug house," so we suspect that such marketing methods were common enough, but on the whole, doctors simply do not tell us about their interactions with pharmaceutical firms or how, once they had gone into practice, they discovered new products or new therapeutic methods.[21] They might purchase medical books and pamphlets, of course, correspond with colleagues, or attend meetings and conferences, but it is most likely that American physicians got their news from medical journals.

Some 250 medical periodicals were founded in the United States between 1797 and 1875 (not including journals that catered to the sects or to pharmacists).[22] Many of these lasted only a short time, and a number were simply forums for the idiosyncratic views of their publishers or editors, or thinly disguised promotions for various manufacturers.[23] But others were sincere attempts to present sound, scientific material, debate professional concerns, and generally contribute to improving the tone of regular medicine.[24] One of their chief functions was to abstract the latest news from Europe or major American centers, so that even doctors on the western frontier were able to keep up to date. Typically, each issue of any journal had at least one feature article of general interest, as well as several communications from ordinary practitioners, who wrote about interesting experiences that might prove helpful to their colleagues. In fact, the periodicals carried a good deal of pharmaceutical information in their text pages—but even more in their advertising pages. Although ethical companies rejected lay advertising, they did not ban publicizing their merchandise to physicians. Virtually all medical journals therefore contained substantial amounts of promotional material from drug companies, in addition to notices from suppliers of the other essential items of the doctor's life: office equipment, medical books, surgical supplies, buggies, malpractice insurance.

In the absence of company records (which either no longer exist or are not often available to outsiders), the surviving journal advertisements give us access to some of the activities of drug companies that might otherwise go unnoticed. The contents and manner of display provide interesting insights, although unfortunately libraries have usually deleted advertising pages when binding the journals, so ads are not always easy to find, especially in situ. Nevertheless, enough remain to confirm that advertisements did indeed play an important role in American medicine.

Before the Civil War, one of the standard methods of pharmaceutical advertising was simply a list of the company's inventory, with or without prices, and usually without any fancy fonts or devices. This plain style was partly the result of limits imposed by printing technology, but it may also have reflected the company's wish to avoid any unfavorable comparisons to nostrum advertisers, who were already making extravagant claims in the nation's newspapers.[25] Yet a large number of ethical manufacturers quickly departed from this sedate mode, creating eye-catching advertisements that could hardly escape notice. After the war this process accelerated, aided by developments in printing and media technology. Illustrations of bottles, labels, medals awarded at trade shows, or elaborate designs and motifs began to appear in the ads. The William R. Warner Company of Philadelphia, whose founder was said to have had a flare for publicity,[26] supplied advertisements to a large number of medical and pharmaceutical journals as four-page leaflets illustrated with such devices, inserted in nearly every issue, often printed on garishly colored paper—bright yellow, hot pink, and

PARKE, DAVIS & CO.,

Manufacturing Chemists,

Laboratory, McDougall Avenue, Guoin and Atwater Streets,
Business Office, No. 52 Larned Street West,

DETROIT, - - - - MICH.

MANUFACTURERS OF

AQUA AMMONIÆ,   CHEM. PURE CHLOROFORM,
SPIRITS NITRE DULC.,   TINC. MUR. IRON, &c.

We make a specialty of the above Chemicals, and can offer them as low as any manufacturers in the country. Western buyers will save time and freight charges by purchasing of us. Send for quotations.

PARKE, DAVIS & CO.'S

Standard Medicinal Fluid and Solid Extracts.

SOLUBLE SUGAR COATED PILLS,

CONCENTRATIONS, ELIXIRS, WINES AND SYRUPS, &c., &c.

We call special attention to the following articles, lately added to our list:

FLUID EXTRACT GUARANA.
FLUID EXTRACT EUCALYPTUS GLOBULES.
FLUID EXTRACT BEARSFOOT.
FLUID EXTRACT CALENDULA.
FLUID EXTRACT CHESTNUT LEAVES.
FLUID EXTRACT CONIUM SEED.
FLUID EXTRACT COTTON ROOT BARK, (from the fresh root.)
FLUID EXTRACT GELSEMINUM, (from the fresh root.)
FLUID EXTRACT STAVESACRE SEED.
PILLS OF PICRATE AMMONIUM, (Sugar Coated.)
BRUNDAGE'S ANTI-CONSTIPATION PILLS, (Sugar Coated.)

Send for dose, descriptive list and circulars, which will be forwarded on application.
Physicians who desire our preparations will please specify P., D. & Co. on their prescriptions.
Our list of manufactures can be obtained of the following Wholesale Druggists, at Manufacturer's rates

R. Macready & Co.,..Cincinnati. O.
Kenyon, Potter & Co.,...Syracuse, N. Y.
Jno. A. Kelly & Co.,...Pittsburg, Pa.
Benton, Myers & Canfield,..Cleveland, O.
Geo. M. Dixon,..Dayton, O.
A. Peter & Co',...Louisville, Ky.
E. Burnham, Son & Co.,..Chicago, Ill.
A. A. Mellier,...St. Louis, Mo.
Colburn, Birks & Co.,..Peoria, Ill.
Geo. A. Eddy,...Leavenworth, Kan.
Godbe & Co.,..Salt Lake City, Utah.
Plain, Williams & Co.,...Toledo, O
Shrewsbury Bros.,...Parkersburg, W. Va.
Farrand, Williams & Co.,...Detroit, Mich.
Swift & Dodds...Detroit, Mich.

DEPOT IN CHICAGO,

E. BURNHAM, SON & CO.

FIGURE 1. An early Parke-Davis ad that is typical of the advertising by ethical firms in that it simply lists the products, most of which are botanicals, but also includes Brundage's Anti-Constipation Pills—a nostrum.

From *New Remedies* (1875).

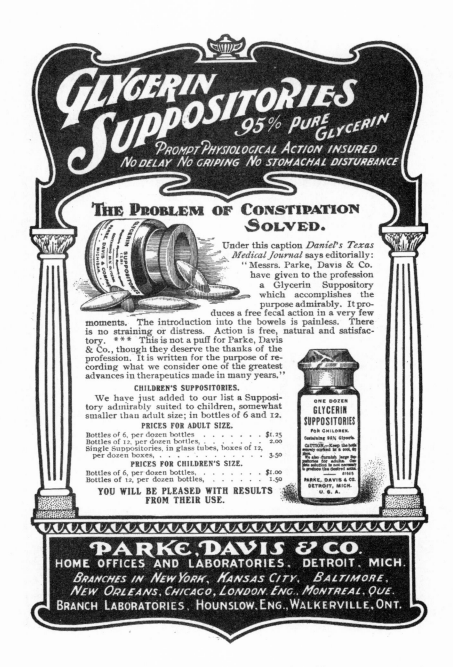

FIGURE 2. By the turn of the century, Parke-Davis's ads had become very attractive and usually appeared in the most desirable locations in the periodical.

From *American Journal of Pharmacy* 73 (November 1901).

mauve were common. Intended to fall out into the reader's lap, these flyers surely must have induced a number of practitioners to consider Warner's products. (And possibly convinced others to reject them, but Warner was a successful company, so presumably the ads had a positive effect over all.) At the end of the century, print advertising had become even more sophisticated, as the exceptionally attractive ads for Parke-Davis demonstrate. Artistic, bold, and quite elegant, they appeared in a wide variety of medical and pharmaceutical publications, often in the most desirable locations—on a cover or opposite the first page of text.

Reformers do not seem to have considered flashy advertising in itself much of a problem, so long as ethical companies directed it only toward professionals—which, on the whole, they did—and of course, so long as they advertised only suitable products (*USP* items, alkaloidal extracts, and a few standard mixtures)—which, however, on the whole, they did not. It is clear that well before the Civil War, many producers had taken considerable liberties in this area, listing not only nonpharmacopeial items but many refined preparations that went beyond what medical purists considered appropriate. By midcentury such manufactured articles dominated the dealers' merchandise. In 1867 the moderately sized B. Keith and Company of New York City advertised fifty-seven powders, eight oils, and thirty-eight concentrated tinctures.[27] The first price list of Eli Lilly and Company of Indianapolis (1876) was twenty-four pages long, with "312 fluidextracts, 189 sugar-coated pills, 199 gelatine-coated, 50 elixirs, 15 syrups, five wines," and several other items.[28] Also in 1876 the larger F. Stearns Company of Detroit had on hand "a full line of Fluid Extracts, Solid Extracts, Resinoids, Oleo Resins, Medicated Syrups, Sugar Coated Pills, Pure Powdered Drugs, Distilled Water, Packed Roots and Herbs, Medicinal Lozenges, Effervescing Granules, Medicated Elixirs, Suppositories, Plasters, Tinctures, [and] Miscellaneous Products." Its catalog that year was 132 pages long, listing "nearly 10,000 items," most of which were "finished."[29] Although such "finished" items were contrary to the ideals of professional prescribing, the convenience of manufacturers' "precisely measured forms" had quickly made them acceptable.[30] From time to time this annoyed the medical purists, but even the reformers might agree that machine-made sugar-coated pills (and capsules and tablets) were a "refinement of civilization," and if from an otherwise reputable firm, they might be as good or better than those made by hand.[31]

More troubling, however, was the profusion of drug mixtures and medleys that combined ingredients to the manufacturer's, not the physician's, specifications. Some of these concoctions were in fact the original "patent medicines" of the seventeenth or eighteenth century: Dover's Powder (powdered ipecacuanha and opium) and Plummer's Pills (calomel and antimony pills), for example. Having quickly passed into the regular medical repertoire, they had long lost any commercial taint and could appear in catalogs under either the inventor's name or the generic designation.[32] Reformers were not as tolerant of these, but at least the recipes were familiar. Yet many companies also advertised a multitude of mixtures that did not have the sanction of either tradition or current authority, with which, presumably, physicians might not be well acquainted. Indeed, with such a dazzling array of medicines in general, how could practitioners choose between any particular products?

Alert to the possibilities, advertisers by the 1860s had begun to provide more than just lists, prices, and the usual guarantees of purity and quality. They also started to include such things as testimonials from eminent physicians or respected medical editors that endorsed either the product or the manufacturer. So a Dr. C. H. Guptill of Maine advertised his own version of an iodo-bromide calcium compound by excerpting a favorable article on the topic from the *American Journal of Medical Science*.[33] The Massachusetts state assayer apparently pronounced Hazard and Caswell's Cod Liver Oil to be the "the best for Foreign or Domestic use"—at least, according to the ad in an 1867 issue of the *New York Medical Journal*. A competitor's advertisement for cod liver oil on the same page, on the other hand, claimed no endorsement but that of time: "It has stood the test of nearly twenty years' experience, and can be relied on in every particular."[34] The 1874 pill list of the Warner Company included a ten-year-old (but apparently still valid) communication from John M. Maisch, a pharmacist in the United States Army, to the effect that Maisch had examined Warner's pills and found them "both perfect and elegant," the company's "practical experience [being] . . . the surest guaranty of their excellence."[35] The fact that by 1874 Maisch was a well-known advocate for scientific and professional pharmacy and the editor of the *American Journal of Pharmacy* was probably not lost on readers. Ethical firms, after all, were supposed to uphold high standards.

Companies therefore also enticed physicians by emphasizing honest "methods of manufacture, intelligently supervised."[36] Hegeman and Company of New York stated that "We make no claim to any secret mode of concentration or Cold Pressing [of our cod liver oil] but warrant it the pure Ol. Morrhuae."[37] Competitors Hazard and Caswell (noting in 1867 that one Professor Parker, who had "tried almost every other manufacturer's Oil," preferred Hegeman's cod liver oil) implied that the reason this oil was so wonderful was because it was "manufactured on the sea-shore from carefully selected, healthy and fresh livers." Nine years later, Parker still preferred it, and the oil, "strictly pure and scientifically prepared," was still being made right on the beach, only this time there was an illustration of a fishing boat accompanying the text.[38] If praising themselves was not enough, firms could also imply that rival products were not merely inferior but were in fact "worthless imitations" that would harm patients.[39] So said the Dundas Dick Company, for example, when it told doctors that if they did not specify "D. D. & Co." capsules of Soft Sandalwood Oil ("sixty Capsules *only*" would cure an unnamed disease, possibly gonorrhea, in a week), they ran the risk of delaying or even preventing a cure.[40] The manufacturers' name in this case was a virtual guarantee of success.

Other companies, mindful of the difficulty prescribers had in getting their patients to take foul-tasting medicines, emphasized not the medical value of their preparations but their elegance. Thus Reed and Carnrick of New York City in 1876 offered a product that had been "originated with the design of furnishing a liquid cathartic remedy that could be prescribed in a palatable form" even to children.[41] Dr. McMunn's Elixir of Opium, touted as "superior to morphine," was probably rather tasty because an elixir by definition contained sugar and about 25 percent alcohol.[42] The allure of such concoctions for prescribers, as well as for patients, should not be underestimated. It was a matter of considerable professional pride for both physicians and pharmacists that medications not be nauseating or repulsive.[43] The fact that manufacturers had also assumed this skill, however, was becoming a matter of some concern.

Even more disturbing were the increasingly frequent references to the diseases and conditions that a given product would treat, even cure. The Warner Company, for instance, recommended its phosphorous and nux vomica compound for "Lapse of Memory, Softening of the Brain, Loss of

Nerve Power, Phthisis, Paralysis, and Impotency." Frederick Stearns of Detroit sold, among other things, "Castanea. Sweet chestnut leaves used in whooping cough." I. O. Woodruff and Company of New York offered "Freligh's Tablets for the Prevention and Cure of Pulmonary Phthisis."[44] Including such information in the ads defied the tenets of professional drug supply. Manufacturers were not supposed to provide solutions to medical problems. Besides, such information could easily make its way to the public (a possibility the Woodruff Company tried to forestall by refusing to send samples to anyone who could not provide proof he was a real doctor.)

A few companies also began inventing names for their articles, despite the general condemnation of this practice. At first, neologisms seem to have been confined to digestive aids and diet products such as the malt preparation Maltine, the pepsin Papoid, and the supplement made from lactated pepsin, Lactopeptine. This last item was introduced in the early 1870s, but its advertising did not indicate that the word itself was a trademark until the 1880s. By then, however, many other coined words were beginning to appear, including Celerina, containing the "nerve-toning principles of celery, coca, and viburnum"; Quinquinia, with four different cinchona alkaloids; Vaseline, petroleum jelly or gelatum petrolei; and Listerine, a liquid antiseptic for internal, external, and oral use. All tried to avoid the appearance of impropriety by including their formulas or ingredients in their advertising and on their labels. Their products came to be known as "ethical proprietaries," but by continuing to disdain public advertising their manufacturers remained within the ethical camp and were persistent in describing themselves as upstanding representatives of the pharmaceutical manufacturing fraternity.

The behavior of these companies may nevertheless have been less than virtuous, however. The advertising of the Stearns Company of Detroit, for example—the very firm that claimed to have invented the concept of the nonsecret formula—named the diseases for which its products could be used, suggesting therapeutic connections that the physician was supposed to make on his own. In fact the owner, Frederick Stearns, had been expelled from the American Pharmaceutical Association (APhA) in 1869 for selling a fraudulent nostrum. He had promoted a "sweet quinine" preparation (quinine was one of the most bitter substances known) that contained cinchonine, not quinine, and was therefore said to be mislabeled. He had even promised to send samples to "those physicians and others wishing to test" the product (noting as well that its name was copyrighted).[45]

Even the company of the exemplary Dr. Edward Squibb, who personally opposed "all forms of copyright and trade-mark and patent from the mildest forms of the manufacture of coated pills to the aggravated abominations of the patent medicine market" (and who had engineered the expulsion of Frederick Stearns from the APhA), was itself not without faults.[46] At least once Squibb was accused of overcharging.[47] Advertisements for Squibb products, however, are difficult to find. This may be an accident of preservation, but it may also be that because Squibb's specialty products (the anesthetics) did not have much competition, they did not require much promotion. Perhaps Squibb could afford to be righteous. Of all ethical companies in the United States, Squibb's remained among the most respected, frequently cited as an example of how a pharmaceutical manufacturer should conduct itself.

Parke, Davis and Company, on the other hand, although it declared that it detested medical patents, commercial secrecy, and monopolies, nevertheless advertised widely and handsomely, and was not at all reluctant to remind physicians that they were merchants: "On a trade basis only do we present ourselves, and to the rules of trade do we conform."[48] Yet as a business engaged in the provision of life-saving or health-giving commodities, Parke-Davis had concerns over and above the merely commercial and took pains to represent itself as fundamentally benevolent and selfless. Interspersed among the usual advertisements for its products were essays on the company's character, which Parke-Davis hoped would inspire physicians to patronize them because of "the integrity of our motives."[49] In 1894, in fact, the company described in detail "the ethical, scientific, and business principles" on which it based its "operations as manufacturing chemists": it was committed to "the highest standard of quality"; it rejected patents, trade marks, and secret formulas; it would not "label or advertise . . . products [so] as to encourage . . . their use by the public without the advice of the physician."[50] The company believed that a worthy formula "should be published in scientific literature in such a manner that any competent pharmacist may readily prepare it." And finally, it believed that manufacturing chemists "ought not to act altogether from a selfish pecuniary motive, but should have in view the general well-being of humanity, and as tending to this end, the continued progress of medicine and pharmacy."[51]

Just how effective the company's advertising was is difficult to judge. At least one doctor praised "the name of P., D., & Co. [as] a synonym for honesty and fair dealing" and was so pleased with its preparations that "even where hope of life [had] almost fled," he felt "fully assured that if there [were] any recuperative power left . . . they [would] aid that power and bring about speedy convalescence." (That this letter was written to the *Therapeutic Gazette*, a Parke-Davis publication, might have had some influence on the author's opinion, however.)[52] At any rate, in its first year of business (1875), net sales amounted to $87,058, and the company did not show a profit until the following year. But in 1885, sales were $942,882 and continued to increase steadily, averaging $3.2 million per year between 1892 and 1901. After 1900 the company claimed to be the world's largest pharmaceutical manufacturer, and still, apparently, one of the world's most ethical, for in 1919 a series of advertisements on "The House with a Policy" ran in various medical journals around the country.[53] Advertising its products as well as its principles must surely have contributed to this success.

At the same time, a growing contingent of physicians was less than pleased with the conspicuously commercial behavior of the ethical drug industry. At the very least the industry was contributing to a prescribing environment that medical reformers found troubling. The AMA considered many of these proprietary items to be inherently deceitful, and its own code of ethics contended that it was "derogatory to professional character" to prescribe or create such things because such actions implied "either disgraceful ignorance or fraudulent avarice."[54] Even companies that were not deceitful about their proprietaries' contents might still be guilty of other misdeeds. Because proprietaries were costlier than generics (that is, *USP* items), customers needed a persuasive reason to buy them. Listerine, therefore, was not just a good antiseptic, or even the best available, but "the most powerful antiseptic and restorative yet discovered."[55] To many observers, ethical proprietaries had come dangerously close to being true nostrums. They had also come dangerously close to being the only kinds of medicines that many post–Civil War American doctors prescribed.

In 1882 Yale professor C. A. Lindsley outlined the disturbing situation in some detail. There was now, he said, "a host of different formulas, some of them of very complex nature and containing some of the most active and potent agents," nicely packaged, but having only one "apology for their existence, that they save[d] the prescriber the trouble of thinking, and relieve[d] the druggist of the exercise of any special knowledge of his business." The use of such readymade articles would diminish "the capacity of making nice therapeutic adaptations of remedies." A popular although nonpharmacopeial concoction of iron, quinine, and strychnine, for example, was supplied by dozens of manufacturers, but each version had a different proportion of ingredients, which the manufacturers could change without notice; indeed, the formulas they supplied in their advertising were "for the most part deceptive." The recipes could not be duplicated.[56] In fact, as the chairman of the New York State Medical Association's committee on legislation complained, some labels identified only the active ingredients. He believed a truly ethical formula would list all of its components.[57]

In the opinion of many reformers, deception or nondisclosure put such articles firmly into the nostrum camp. Although other commercialisms might be forgiven if the product was in some way useful, secrecy of any kind was utterly contrary to professional ideals. If we use these articles, said the *Medical Record*, "how can we reconcile our pretentious advocacy of the claims of scientific medicine? The use of secret remedies is such a disgraceful reflection upon the resources of our art, that the best we can say for it is that the more the practice is hidden in the humiliation of our own incompetency the better for the profession at large."[58] Medical men used to have a position of trust in the community, said a Massachusetts physician, but now the public could not tell the difference between a real doctor and a quack.[59]

Secrecy or obfuscation also resulted from the increasing use of trade names. Drug names were supposed to be scientific and relate to the chemistry of the item, but, as Lindsley asked, what was to be made of "Lactopeptine? Maltine? Vitalized-Phosphate? Celerina? . . . Hydroleine? Listerine? . . . and a more innumerable host of mixtures?" They were "inventions of tradesmen, and in no sense represent[ed] the growth and progress of medical science." "What pretensions [could] physicians make to scientific practice whose therapeutics [were] based on such unstable foundations?" These articles had "no vitality other than what they derive[d] from the advertising pages." It was the same as using Hop Bitters or Swain's Panacea.[60]

Although the "better" class of medical proprietaries was sold only to medical men, said Lindsley, advertisements for them were as gaudy as those for the cure-alls and had the same enthusiastic testimonials. These testimonials, however, were not from satisfied patients but from "*teachers! Mirabile dictu!* teachers of medicine! Heaven help their students, and their future patients, if this is the sort of therapeutics taught in the colleges these professors represent." Moreover, professional proprietaries had a marketing feature the nostrums did not—the detailman (the trade's term for salesman). "Our offices," he said, "are daily beset with polite, well-dressed and loquacious emissaries" of pharmaceutical houses, replete with sample cases, who made "dupes of doctors almost as easily as of their patients."[61] An article in the *New York Times* agreed:

> The credulity of some physicians is beyond belief. . . . It is a com-
> plete counterpart . . . to that of the lay public. . . . The agent of a
> manufacturer of some particular preparation calls on a physician
> and assures him that the preparation will cure and has cured the
> most obstinate cases of this and is useful in that, and so on. Without
> further knowledge than this the physician commences to prescribe
> its use. There is unquestionably among an increasing number of
> doctors a tendency to avoid the writing of prescriptions, and
> depend upon ready-made compounds.[62]

This was both unethical and unsafe. Physicians "trusted" that the claimed ingredients were in fact present in the proprietary.

The sophistication of the proprietary manufacturer was not to be admired and applauded but feared, said yet another Massachusetts practitioner. Detailmen visited doctors in their offices, proffering goods with plausible explanations for their use and glowing accounts of their successful application. Doctors were flattered by the attention and the free samples. At some point the salesman might ask for a product endorsement, which was then printed up and circulated, further legitimizing the item.[63] By the late 1880s, according to one observer, there were about 160 manufacturers in the United States "who in reality, for the most part, [were] but mere manipulators and mixers of drugs." In New York City alone, he said, forty companies produced a total of 36,500 mixtures, each with its own name and each "directly at variance with scientific progress" in that the mixtures were neither useful nor innovative.[64]

Yet some practitioners believed it was perfectly responsible to pre-scribe such items if it was in the best interests of the patient.[65] As early as the mid-1870s, the surgeon J. Marion Sims had suggested that because the use of proprietaries was so widespread, the AMA's code of ethics should be updated to accommodate modern practice.[66] (The code, however, made no such concessions at that time.) Nor should the profession reject advertised medicines out of hand: "It would be as untrue as unjust to accuse all our largest drug manufacturers of fostering [irresponsible advertising] . . . since many of these supply to the profession, carefully prepared drugs in such pure, convenient and palatable forms, as to make them a boon to both physician and patient."[67] A great deal of skill went into a good medi-cine, said an Alabama county health officer. Conscientious manufacturers attempted to standardize their products and meet pharmacopeial require-ments. In his opinion, "not ten percent of the country's physicians" could prescribe such items properly on their own.[68] Even the AMA's own publi-cation (*JAMA*) had to concede that some products had merit.[69] Nonethe-less, most reformers thought that at the very least, all such preparations "should be subject to supervision and regulation," presumably by regular medical men.[70] A New York practitioner simply proposed that the industry police itself by weeding out the dishonest and fraudulent companies, thus enhancing the reputation of legitimate manufacturers.[71]

In general, observers agreed that a doctor should write prescriptions "from his brain [and] . . . not resort 'as a cloak for ignorance,' or laziness, to this wholesale prescribing of manufactured medicines."[72] But it is rare to find an offending manufactured concoction actually identified by name in any of the disapproving remarks in the medical journals. The periodicals, in fact, were faced with a dilemma. Most could not survive without the advertising revenue that came from the manufacturers of many of the items being criticized.[73] An editorial in the *Therapeutic Gazette* (by Mr. Davis of Parke-Davis) noted the general fear "that the manufacturers of elegant phar-maceutical preparations and specialties [would] agree to withdraw their advertising patronage from such journals as assail[ed] their interests."[74]

JAMA addressed the problem more directly than most of the other journals did, and in fact its first volume (1883) published a letter from Iowa doctor G. R. Henry critical of Parke-Davis concoctions. "They have taken the place of Ayer's Pectoral and Humboldt's Buchu, and are patronized by all the quacks and all the patent medicine men in this country," said Henry. *JAMA* agreed and lamented that a "well-known firm . . . [had] yielded to the pernicious practice . . . of putting up and selling ready-made prescriptions or formulae" but was grateful that Parke-Davis at least abstained from "the still more objectionable practice of resorting to *trade-mark, copyright,* or other means of holding exclusive proprietorship in medicines of any kind."[75] *JAMA*'s own rules excluded advertisements of items with such unacceptable features, but its membership fees could make up the lost revenue. Other journals also tried to publicize only "recognized preparations" and to limit the number of pages devoted to advertising, but the majority of medical publications had far fewer text pages than those consigned to product promotion.[76] The *Cincinnati Lancet-Clinic* was not so sure that limiting advertisements was such a good idea. High revenue could improve services to readers, as exemplified by the *New York Herald.* This newspaper paid for its good-quality reading matter from its advertising revenues. The British *Lancet* was the largest and best medical journal in the world, and had the highest proportion of advertising pages to text pages of any of them—an average of 32 text and 48 advertising pages per issue. So long as text was not reduced to accommodate the advertisements, ethics were not compromised.[77]

Yet to the AMA and other reform-minded physicians just before the turn of the century, the readymade specialties and ethical proprietaries were persistent, embarrassing evidence of the deficiencies of American medical education and practice. Too many diagnoses were "largely guided by the tablets or pills that the practitioner [happened] to have in stock."[78] One critic estimated that more than one-third of prescriptions were incorrectly written, calling for incompatible ingredients; being ignorant of proper practice, doctors (especially younger ones) favored the proprietaries.[79] Because the profession was not teaching its members, the advertising literature was doing it instead. Commercial interests were dominant because too many physicians were dupes—because they loved to be duped.[80] There were even companies that at one time had sold nostrums to the public but now found it more profitable to market to "reputable though foolish physicians."[81] If practitioners were not careful, manufacturing chemists would soon take over therapeutics. Medical journals collabo-

rated with the drug trade by featuring "original" articles about proprietaries, sometimes with editorial endorsements.[82] The *American Medical
Quarterly*, for example, noted sadly that "so many practitioners" were
impressed with a new drug "solely upon the statements of its manufacturers."[83] Even companies with good products were at fault, especially when
being seen as scientific became an important selling point:

> The clever manufacturers employ able men of science to test with
> care the physiologic and therapeutic actions of their drugs, and
> these reports, when given to us in full, are of genuine value. In sub-
> sequent advertising, however, the results obtained are summarized
> and often so skillfully that disagreeable effects are lost sight of or
> minimized. Moreover, these summaries are imbedded in a mass of
> optimistic writing by the advertiser or by physicians who record
> their impressions; not observations made with the accuracy which
> science demands.
>
> Therefore, even the best of this printed matter, of which we all
> receive so much, is not to be trusted.[84]

All in all, physicians devoted "too little study to materia medica and therapeutics."[85] Advertising was becoming their chief source of information. Yet
critics of proprietaries—especially the AMA and other reformers who were
keenly aware of the need for physicians to be acquainted with contemporary progress in science if they wanted their status to improve—constantly
emphasized that there was no good reason for any doctor to prescribe any
drug that possessed any commercial features whatsoever. Every ingredient, compound, and recipe that could be used in rational, scientific medical practice consisted of items that were in the public domain. The
solution to proprietary prescribing was well within the grasp of the profession so long as the will was there.[86]

There was, however, a small cloud on the horizon. Some of the very
items that European science had recently produced, whose use in prescriptions could potentially enhance the image of the physician as up to
date, well informed, and accomplished, were about to make it difficult for
American doctors to prescribe both scientifically and noncommercially.
German synthetic drugs were poised to turn the medical world on its ear.

And headaches at long last were about to obtain some relief.

4

The Remarkable Synthetic Drugs

In the spring of 1856, an English teenager, home for Easter from the Royal College in London where he was studying chemistry, spent his vacation experimenting with aniline, a chemical found in coal tar. Coal tar was an abundant but otherwise fairly useless waste product of the illuminating gas industry, which chemists nevertheless found interesting because of the variety of organic compounds they could make from it. The young Englishman was hoping to create artificial quinine. But instead of the drug, he produced a purple dye. He immediately quit school and took out a patent on his discovery. In the following year, a young French chemistry professor published the first in a series of papers claiming that fermentation (such as occurs when grape juice becomes wine or wine becomes vinegar) was caused by microscopic organisms. He caught the attention of the French wine industry, although his ideas were only of marginal interest to anyone else—at least at first. But within thirty years, these two apparently unrelated events would converge in unanticipated ways, with considerable implications for medicine in general and for the headache in particular.

When young William Henry Perkin realized he had created a dyestuff instead of a drug, he at once saw its commercial possibilities and by 1857 was running a factory whose only product was that purple dye, aniline mauve. He quickly became a millionaire. Before he retired from business at the ripe old age of thirty-six to again devote himself to pure research, Perkin had discovered a few more dyes, had developed a few more industrial processes, and was credited with founding the modern organic chemical industry. By the time of his death in 1908, this industry was producing not only synthetic dyestuffs but preservatives, fertilizers, perfumes, artificial flavorings, high explosives—and medicines, as we shall see. The material world would never again be the same.[1]

Meanwhile, Louis Pasteur's thesis that microorganisms caused fermentation had grown into the germ theory of disease, an exciting but controversial topic that was widely debated by the late 1870s.[2] To its opponents, the theory relied too much on the mysterious, vital forces of mysterious, elusive bacteria and was asking medicine to return to an era of vague and imprecise speculation just when the materialism of physics and chemistry was providing some measure of certainty. To its supporters, however, germ theory had at least two significant advantages. First, bacteria were not mystical forces but real entities that could be seen and studied in the laboratory (indeed, they could be most easily seen when stained with one of the new synthetic dyestuffs), making it both possible and likely that their role in disease would be determined with scientific precision. And second, bacteria offered immediate therapeutic possibilities. Because they were specific, physical *things*, specific physical antidotes or cures might be found—a prospect that delighted contemporaries who thought this would finally allow "the practice of medicine [to] take its place among the sciences which are called exact."[3] Even more consequential was the fact that microbes were alive. It was as *living* organisms that they were dangerous. (Dead, in fact, they were helpful, because as Pasteur had discovered, inoculation with dead or weakened germs became the principle of immunization.) So germ theorists proposed that the most direct way to deal with bacteria was to kill or cripple them. The British surgeon Joseph Lister had based his antiseptic techniques on this premise, using phenol (carbolic acid, also derived from coal tar) as his germ killer to prevent wound infection. His spectacular results became well known, arousing a great deal of hopeful expectation that antisepsis might also work *inside* the body.[4] Phenol, unfortunately, had no virtue as an internal germ killer. It is highly poisonous and used internally would be as harmful to patients as to microscopic life. It was disease prevention (immunity induced by inoculation) rather than cure that actually gave germ theory its first great successes. Internal germ killers and specific antimicrobial "antidotes" would not be discovered for several more decades.

Germ theory, however, was of course not the only topic that medical science explored in the nineteenth century. By the time Pasteur published his first essays on fermentation, investigators had already been employing some of the innovative mechanistic concepts being developed in physiology and pathology to study one of the most pressing concerns of the medical world—fevers, with results that would prove significant for many aspects of medicine in general and, in a roundabout way, for headache in particular. *Fever* was a term used for centuries to identify diseases characterized by a collection of acute symptoms, high temperature (pyrexia) being the most distinctive (headaches, of course, often being present as well). Because the vast majority of dangerous ailments and epidemics were febrile, physicians generally welcomed any progress in the understanding of the processes of both normal and abnormal body temperature. By about 1860, in fact, most physicians were satisfied that animal heat was not a metaphysical vital force but a quantifiable physio-chemical one, a form of oxidation, and probably regulated by the central nervous system. Somehow this malfunctioned in fevers, producing the characteristic heat.[5]

At the same time, researchers were also studying putrefaction and fermentation, which likewise produce heat, and which were thought to be analogous to febrile processes. Most scientists were confident that all these phenomena would turn out to be physical or chemical in nature and would vindicate mechanistic approaches to vital functions—that is, until Pasteur and other germ theorists suggested that microscopic life forms might play an important role and thus threw the whole business into turmoil. Germ theory became more acceptable, however, when it was conceded that bacteria did not operate only as living organisms but also as physical beings with chemical properties; the mechanistic and vital approaches to disease causation and pathology were therefore not mutually incompatible. Thus, over the last quarter of the nineteenth century, medical science used these new concepts to reshape, even eradicate, centuries of medical wisdom, replacing the essentially vitalistic traditions of constitutionalism and holism with "recognizably modern notions of specific, mechanism-based ailments with characteristic clinical courses."[6]

Fever studies also had a significant impact on therapeutic practices. Although some physicians believed high temperatures could be beneficial, most researchers were convinced that fevers over 40°C (104°F) were deleterious, and they provided clinical statistics and experimental laboratory results to make their case. The corollary of their findings was that efforts to reduce febrile temperature (antipyresis) produced better outcomes—measurably (that is, scientifically) so, in their opinions. This frankly symptomatic treatment—most often achieved with cold water—made some physicians uncomfortable (although not nearly so uncomfortable as the hapless patients who were forced to endure it), but its adoption gave physicians a sense of control in the face of serious illness and was an energetic example of the activity that defined their professional identity.[7]

Supporters of these symptomatic measures met the charge of empiricism by linking the therapy to their theories of febrile processes, for, as it turned out, antipyresis was not simply a matter of cooling down a hot body with a cold bath. The phenomena were more complex than that. Quinine, for example, was also observed to reduce temperatures, especially in malaria, and no one supposed that it acted like cold water.[8] Instead, quinine's actions were increasingly explained in terms of its ability to inhibit oxidation at the cellular level and thus reduce temperature.[9] Germ theorists also hopefully identified quinine as a possible internal antiseptic or germ killer, one of the causes of high temperature now being ascribed to bacteria. In nonmalarial fevers, however, quinine was less effective, and its antiseptic qualities were quickly doubted, but it was nonetheless widely employed, despite its many side effects and its expense.[10] A cheaper synthetic version had long been very desirable and was one of the reasons young Mr. Perkin became busy in the spring of 1856. The discovery of aniline mauve sidetracked him, but other investigators continued the hunt.

The synthesis of organic chemicals from coal tar in fact proceeded at a furious pace in the second half of the nineteenth century, although it was the search for dyestuffs that commanded most attention. But it was no longer a search that the British led. By the 1880s, German firms produced the majority of the world's artificial dyes and related chemicals. Supported by government, banks, and the universities, the German chemical companies had been part of the newly united Reich's attempt to become a Great Power, and other nations quickly conceded that the Germans had no equals as industrial organic chemists. Appreciated for their excellent dyestuffs, they were also noted for their astute—some would say ruthless—business practices, including a tenacious hold on intellectual property.

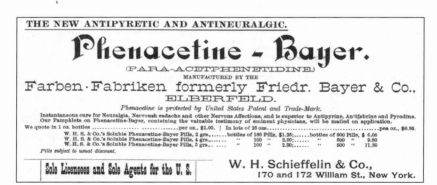

FIGURE 3. A typical Bayer ad in which both Bayer and the trade names were emphasized. In this case, the chemical name of Phenacetin is also supplied, reinforcing the
proprietary nature of the trade name after the expiration of the patent.

From *Pharmaceutical Era* (1917).

Because German chemical patent laws were the most stringent anywhere,
by international agreement a German patent was honored all over the
world, saving the inventor a considerable amount of bother. But although
the strict requirements meant that many chemicals were never awarded
German protection, the inventors could still obtain monopoly rights in
other countries. German firms therefore became masterly managers of the
patent laws of the world, a crucial factor in their control of the industry.[11]

In most countries, a patent was intended to provide an inventor with
a short-term monopoly (seventeen years in the United States) as a reward
for his ingenuity. In the volatile world of textile dyes, a color might become
unfashionable or a process obsolete long before the patent expired, so the
patent was no guarantee of profits. Moreover, in most jurisdictions, only
the manufacturing process, as distinct from the product, could usually
obtain this protection. The chemical itself was in the public domain, and
any manufacturer was free to make it by another method. But even a brief
monopoly could allow the manufacturer to recoup some costs, so Germans
patented their products whenever and wherever they could, vigorously
prosecuting infringers and imitators wherever they encountered them.[12]
Such pugnacity was nothing new to Americans. In the United States, the
virtues of patents and the disputes that arose because of them were
already a part of the business environment, brought to public attention
when famous inventors such as Samuel Morse and Thomas Edison

defended their property rights in court. Industrial patents in themselves were not immoral. Indeed, they were just common sense. But as we have already noted, the status of a medicinal patent was far less exalted. American medical and scientific professionals had declared themselves to be on the side of the angels. It was dishonorable to hold suffering humanity hostage to the greed implied by a patent. The Germans, as acknowledged world leaders in medical and chemical sciences, must surely subscribe to the same high principles. A medical patent was simply unthinkable.

In Germany, however, academic chemistry had developed within a university system that fostered a closer alliance between scholars and commerce than existed elsewhere.[13] German professors were encouraged to patent their discoveries and to sell or license them to firms that could exploit them. The name of Justus Liebig, for example, Germany's preeminent organic chemist, appeared on the label of a nutritional supplement, with his blessing (and apparently to the increase of his personal fortune). In fact, the reputation of German chemists was such that for many years Liebig's Extract was not considered to be a proprietary medicine in the way that Dr. McMunn's Elixir of Opium was. All companies used university professors as their de facto researchers, even after the firms had established their own research departments and had hired staff chemists. It was this academic connection that had earned the German dye industry its reputation as a respectable, science-based enterprise. That it was also highly competitive went with the territory, and the industry made no apology for its commercial features. No one expected it to. So long as the companies and chemistry professors confined themselves to dyestuffs and similar items, commerce and conscience did not clash. In the mid-1880s, however, this was to change when industrial chemistry began to produce coal tar substances with medical applications.

The seeds of this connection were actually planted in 1874 when Hermann Kolbe, the professor of chemistry at Leipzig University, inspired by the current debates about germ theory, announced he had synthesized an *internal* antiseptic.[14] He had created salicylic acid—a compound found naturally in willow trees (*Salix alba*) and other plants—from phenol.[15] Kolbe was convinced that salicylic acid was a medical marvel—a panacea, in fact—and suggested it be used to treat all manner of illnesses. Doctors obliged, and for a short time the acid and its salt (sodium salicylate, which was the form more commonly employed) did appear to be wonder drugs. The medical world, however, to its great disappointment, quickly found that the salicylates did not cure any of the diseases for which internal antisepsis had been postulated, although doctors did note a redeeming feature: in acute rheumatism (rheumatic fever) the new drugs lowered temperatures, reduced swelling and inflammation, and in general alleviated this painful and debilitating condition very quickly.[16] The drugs also proved to be very irritating to the stomach and had to be used with considerable caution. Some practitioners shunned them altogether. Indeed, some patients simply refused to take them. Nonetheless, the salicylates were firmly established in medical practice within two or three years of their introduction, documented, and studied all around the world.[17] Even though they cured nothing, and their mode of action was not well understood, they were evidence that hope in science-based therapies was not misplaced. *Scientific American* even went so far as to call salicylic acid "the most important . . . antipyretic ever discovered."[18] The chemicals did not, however, enter medical practice as an act of charity.

One of the reasons Kolbe had first become interested in salicylic acid was because his synthesis could produce large amounts of it efficiently and cheaply. Even before publishing his findings, he had helped to establish a factory, and he remained a silent partner of sorts in the Chemische Fabrik von Heyden for the rest of his life, a connection that made him wealthy.[19] Kolbe had also obtained patents on his production process in every country he could, including the United States. Thus, from the very beginning, salicylic acid violated American medical ethics. Yet it was treated by both its manufacturers and purchasers as an exemplary ethical pharmaceutical item (probably because the acid was already a known chemical and the patent did not prevent access to nonsynthetic versions).

Indeed, except for the patent, salicylic acid lacked any other proprietary features. It was a single chemical compound, not a mixture, and its identity and purity could be easily assayed. Manufactured under stringent conditions as laid out in the patent, its uniformity and potency were constant, so its effects could be anticipated. It could be administered in precise doses. It had no trade name, it was not advertised to the public, and it was only available as a raw powder, which was generally unsuitable for self-medication. Patients almost always obtained it in prescriptions (although there is some evidence that salicylic acid was "common in the preparation of remedies for rheumatism" with which patients were treating themselves).[20] With competitive, non-Kolbe acid also available, prescribers and dispensers were free to make choices based on quality, price, and other criteria. There was no monopoly, no secrecy, and no advertising hyperbole. Advertising copy for the Heyden Company was simply the name of the firm and the chemicals it manufactured. Promotion, such as it was, seems genuinely to have been the good press the drugs received in medical journals.

Early "salicylmania," nevertheless, had cooled a great deal by the mid-1880s, but as antirheumatics, the salicylates were considered very valuable specifics, clear evidence that empirical treatment was no longer always considered to be unprofessional and that drugs could be used to good effect even when they did not fit into the conventional therapeutic categories. Thus for doctors, salicylic acid and sodium salicylate remained very popular antirheumatics, their side effects notwithstanding.[21] Although salicylates were profitable enough for the specialized Heyden Company, their success did not immediately suggest to the larger chemical manufacturers—the source of most of the raw materials—that synthetic medicines ought to become a part of their own business too. Nonetheless, in 1883 the Frankfurt company Farbwerke Meister, Lucius, & Bruning (known as Hoechst), one of Germany's largest dye works, decided to create a pharmaceutical division.[22]

Meanwhile, the search for artificial quinine had never been abandoned. A chemist at the University of Erlangen, Otto Fischer, in 1882 had synthesized a chemical sufficiently related to quinoline (itself a derivative of quinine) to suggest that it might be useful in treating fevers. As was by now the habit of most German chemists, Fischer immediately obtained a patent for it, and after having Erlangen's pharmacologist, Wilhelm Filehne, confirm the chemical's antipyretic properties, he brought the item to the attention of Hoechst. Hoechst was sufficiently impressed to then manufacture and market the drug under a name that Filehne himself had chosen—Kairin (from the Greek for "timely"), a word quite unrelated to the item's chemical designation, hydrochloride of hydroxy-N-ethyltetrahydroquinoline.[23] It flourished briefly as an antipyretic but quickly proved to be too toxic for ordinary fevers and never became popular.[24] The fact that the drug was unethical because it had a patent and a trade name, and that it posed a nomenclature problem in having an impossible "real" name, did not at this time trouble the American medical profession to any degree. Still, the *Druggists Circular* of New York did call attention to the patent and informed its readers that a twenty-gram bottle of Kairin cost $5.00—a very high price.[25] Never used much itself, Kairin nonetheless foreshadowed what was to come. Between 1884 and 1887, the German organic chemical industry introduced three more synthetic antipyretics—Antipyrine, Antifebrin, and Phenacetin—all of which were to have a profound impact on contemporary medical practice.

Until the arrival of synthetics, virtually any new drug that was introduced was closely related to medicines already in use, and therefore the pharmacological properties of the new drug could be anticipated with some certainty. Practitioners were notified of new items (or new combinations or new applications) in communications ranging from letters to the editor of a minor periodical, to an increasing number of sophisticated hospital-based studies conducted by leading (often German) physicians and pharmacologists, accompanied by chemical analyses and other trappings of up-to-date science, published in the leading medical journals, and abstracted in many others. Our modern concepts of drug evaluations, however (statistical analysis, large numbers of patients, randomized, double-blind trials, and so on), were still in the future. In the nineteenth century, all new medicines were really tested only in practice, on real patients in real conditions.[26] An important therapeutic innovation might just as easily appear in a letter to the editor of a local medical paper as in a peer-reviewed article in a prestigious journal.

In most cases, readers of these communications learned of the drug's actions, the recommended doses, what side effects were observed, and whether men, women, or children reacted differently. If the outcome was encouraging, the author invited other doctors to try the drug on their own patients. Adverse reactions would be reported as they occurred, and if they were too frequent and too excessive, use of the drug would largely stop, as had been the case with Kairin.[27] Scientific medicine may have created new disease models and made specifics more respectable, but it had not yet eradicated patient individuality or the doctor's judgment. It was a physician's professional obligation to learn about new remedial agents; it was his professional privilege to determine how, when, or if these agents should be used on his own patients. Medicine at the bedside was still very much an art. And as far as the American medical elite were concerned, it went without saying that any new drug that hoped to gain favor with professionals would be assiduously ethical—that is, a public domain item with a Latin or public name, competitively available from any number of drug companies, and never advertised to laymen.

The synthetic antipyretics did not at first appear to violate these principles in any obvious way and indeed improved on them, with their German origins helping to enhance their reputations as state-of-the-art medications. Antipyrine, for example (like Kairin, the result of collaboration between researchers at the University of Erlangen and Hoechst), was introduced by Wilhelm Filehne only after laboratory analysis and tests on animals and "on healthy and on several feverish people." But Filehne had nevertheless anticipated that the chemical would be an antipyretic because of its supposed relationship to the botanical quinoline. So, encouraged by the initial findings, he sent the chemical to three hospitals, where it was used on an unstated number of fever patients, both adults and children, for about three months. Although the effective doses were high and the results not consistent (some patients needed more medicine, or the temperature reduction did not last very long), side effects were negligible (some vomiting) and the author was optimistic. Filehne's brief publication in 1884 announcing these findings also noted that the drug was not yet available for general use and that the manufacturer would only supply enough for more clinical tests in a hospital setting. This implied that scientific honesty and professional integrity were uppermost for Hoechst and Filehne both, despite the fact that Filehne did not fully identify the chemical he was introducing. He called it only Antipyrine, promising a fuller description in a later communication. The name Antipyrine was of course immediately suggestive of the chief property of the drug, and physicians around the world clamored to try it on their febrile patients. By the end of 1884 there were more than forty publications describing various clinical experiences, including one or two by American doctors. Most reports were positive, but there was no apparent censorship of negative results. The medical press published what doctors reported; other physicians could assess the information as they saw fit.[28]

As with any other new, ethical medication, doctors learned about Antipyrine primarily from the pages of legitimate professional journals. Howard Culbertson, for example, an Ohio practitioner, said he found out about this drug by reading the August 1884 number of the *Boston Medical [and Surgical] Journal*. His references to almost all the current literature suggest he had a methodical way of informing himself and had become thoroughly acquainted with the drug's applications and idiosyncrasies even before he used it in his own practice.[29] In December an army doctor, noting that Antipyrine had "riveted the attention of the most prominent German physicians during the past summer," also noted that "the experimental state is evidently past and nothing but a large number of clinical observations is needed to define absolutely the range of its usefulness." After his own good results, he encouraged other physicians to give the drug a try.[30] His recommendation was scarcely needed, however, for by the time his article appeared, Antipyrine was already being used in the United States to such an extent that it had become scarce, "the manufacturers in Germany not being able to supply the demand."[31] So exciting did this new substance become that even the *New York Times* effusively declared that "Among the many remedies that have been discovered to alleviate the ills of suffering humanity none is more important than Antipyrine." As a fever agent it was probably more effective and less dangerous than other febrifuges, including cold water, and "has received the indorsement of, and is used by the leading practitioners in this country and abroad, and also in all the hospitals of this city." (The newspaper reminded readers, however, that "Antipyrine does not claim to cure a disease, it simply reduces temperature.")[32]

The introduction of the other two synthetics eased the demand on Antipyrine by providing competition. Kalle and Company, a fairly small firm, launched Antifebrin in 1886;[33] Farbenfabriken Bayer, a very large firm located in Elberfeld near Frankfurt on the Rhine, brought a related chemical, Phenacetin, to market the next year.[34] These, too, proved to be excellent antipyretics, but because they were not identical in speed of action or duration of effects, they gave practitioners a choice, based on the needs of the case. Even such a famous therapeutic skeptic as William Osler admitted that he sometimes found Antifebrin useful.[35] The drugs were exactly what the medical profession had hoped science would provide: experimentally and clinically evaluated ethical medications to be used according to the doctor's judgment. The drugs also benefited from what industry could provide: consistent, pure products made to exacting specifications. The synthetics were not without their hazards, however, and some physicians declined to use them at all because their side effects were bizarre and unexpected (allegedly coloring patients blue, for example).[36] "Depressing the heart"—a rather imprecise concept associated with circulatory collapse and general prostration—was the most serious problem associated with them, but despite a small core of critics who considered them too toxic, the synthetic antipyretics became established in the medical repertoire almost immediately and were listed in the catalogs of all the major jobbers.

At $1.25 to $1.30 an ounce in the United States, Antipyrine and Phenacetin were about twice as expensive as quinine sulphate but were used in much smaller doses. Costing even less was Kalle's Antifebrin, available for only twenty-five cents an ounce. This large price difference was not, however, the result of Kalle's wish to make an important new medicine affordable; nor was it because Kalle's product was "cheap," since Antifebrin was regarded as a high-quality drug. Rather, Antifebrin cost so much less because, unlike its competitors, it did not possess a U.S. patent. Antipyrine and Phenacetin only had to compete with each other, not with generic versions of themselves. Antifebrin, on the other hand, was also available as acetanilid and was sold by other German and Swiss firms for only about ten cents an ounce.[37] Even so, Kalle still made a profit, because its product possessed a commercial feature even more valuable than a patent—the name Antifebrin. Rarely did doctors use the generic acetanilid. They almost always wrote "Antifebrin" on their prescription orders, in which case pharmacists were obligated to dispense the brand-name product, because Kalle could sue them for violating the company's property rights if they dispensed any other manufacturer's item.

The names of all three synthetics, in fact, were trade names, owned as private property by their manufacturers, a commercialism that, along with the two patents, did not go unremarked. These drugs "come to us covered all over with patents," lamented the *National Druggist.* "In a word, they are patent medicines in the widest and strictest sense of the term."[38] It was indeed regrettable, said the *Boston Medical and Surgical Journal,* "that

[Antipyrine's] originator should not have felt it unworthy of German science to cover the discovery with a patent,"[39] although some observers pointed out that in the case of these artificial medicines, a patent might not be such a bad thing. Patent documents would reveal the complete production process, and no secrecy would obscure the true nature of drugs that were not analogs of any botanical substance and hence were terra incognita for most doctors. A single manufacturer also could guarantee a consistent product.[40] The chief problem, however, was that while the patent was in force, its owner could charge any price at all: "A large demand will, of course, lessen the expense of production, but as a monopoly will exist . . . the price can be artificially maintained."[41] Indeed, until the U.S. patent expired, the wholesale price for Antipyrine in the United States always ranged between $1.25 and $1.40 per ounce. (By comparison, quinine sulphate was about sixty to seventy-five cents per ounce, and the salicylates about $2.00 per pound.) In 1900, two years after the U.S. patent's expiration, Hoechst's Antipyrine cost a mere thirty-one cents per ounce. Antifebrin, already cheap to start with, cost only fifty cents a pound by 1896, further evidence to the critics of medicinal patents that the monopolies granted to acetanilid's cousins kept prices artificially high and were detrimental to the public welfare.[42]

Patents at least had the virtue of being limited to seventeen years. Trade names, on the other hand, could potentially remain private property forever.[43] This posed no difficulty if the branded item also had an acceptable generic or "real" name—but this was not the case with all the coal tar drugs. Kairin was the first synthetic antipyretic to illustrate the problem: its proper chemical designation was simply too impractical to use, but *kairin* was completely meaningless as a chemical term. Furthermore, the medical profession's ignorance of organic chemistry meant that when scientific names were provided, physicians were not necessarily enlightened.[44] Uncertain of the chemical terms, doctors preferred the simple, memorable trade name, despite complaints from reformers that this amounted to prescribing unknown substances and was therefore unprofessional. The reformers had originally aimed their criticisms at the obfuscations of the proprietary trade. To find that these new marvels of pharmaceutical science were similarly deceptive was a constant source of annoyance to many physicians, although it is apparent that initially, the rank and file were not altogether aware that a problem existed. Doctors had considered Kairin, for example, simply a convenient synonym for the scientific term, much as they might write "laudanum" instead of "tincture of opium." Kairin's rapid journey into neglect prevented any difficulties arising from this situation. Antipyrine, on the other hand, remained popular long enough to reveal just what these issues were.

Because the name Antipyrine was owned by Hoechst, it could be used only to refer to Hoechst's product. Rival manufacturers would have to call their versions something else. (Rival versions, of course, were moot until the patent expired, this being the one synthetic antipyretic that was novel enough for even the German courts to reward with a monopoly.) Moreover, the name deliberately evoked the idea of antipyresis and suggested nothing about the drug's chemical constitution. Critics complained that this might lead practitioners to consider the drug only for use as a febrifuge, ignoring any other properties it might have. Instead of leaving the therapeutic decisions to practitioners, such unscientific nomenclature subtly sought to teach doctors when and why the product should be employed. This was a characteristic of proprietary, not professional, drugs. Filehne himself had been unhappy about the choice of the name Antipyrine. Early in 1884 he wrote to the head of Hoechst's pharmaceutical division that this was "a secretive sounding name. It is far too reminiscent of 'Anodyne,' 'Antihydropin' and similar dubious items." He wanted something "more neutral . . . which does not relate to the drug's effect" and suggested "quinizine . . . knorrine or hoechstine." Calling it Antipyrine, he said, "would discredit the substance in the face of science." Because his introductory article was to be published without the details of the drug's constitution, it was all the more important, he said, to avoid the appearance of impropriety. If Hoechst went ahead with the name as planned, Filehne wanted everyone to know that the choice went against his wishes.[45] (It seems, however, that the rest of the world believed that the "deceptive but enticing name 'Antipyrin'" was indeed Filehne's invention.)[46]

The trade name might not have been so troublesome, however, if a convenient chemical synonym (that is, a public name) had also been made available. But Filehne's first publication in 1884 referred only to Antipyrin, intimating that the new drug was related to quinoline in some way but leaving Ludwig Knorr, the Erlangen chemist who was the actual inventor, to eventually publish the details of the composition in literature not normally read by the medical profession, at least not in the United States.[47] In an article appearing later that year (which noted that the substance was already being used in medical practice as Antipyrine), Knorr identified his discovery as methyloxyquinizine, which modern chemists renamed hydroxymethylquinizine.[48] Knorr's substance actually was phenyldimethylpyrazolone, from a quite different class of organic chemicals, which Knorr must have already known, because his patent application the previous year was for "Darstellung von Oxypyrazolen."[49] For the vast majority of practitioners, however, it was the chemical's supposed connection to quinine that gave it legitimacy. With Kairin, a genuine quinoline derivative, doctors had been enticed by an antipyretic that was simply too toxic to use safely, but one that had at least suggested a better version could be found. Antipyrine appeared to be a likely candidate.[50] A "pyrazolone" compound in this context would have been meaningless; a "quinoline" derivative was not. Presumably this is one reason the original publication did not reveal the proper constitution of the drug. Once Antipyrine was well established in medical practice, its identity was no longer a problem, and pyrazolones themselves were investigated further for their medicinal properties.[51] But uncertainty about its true nature nevertheless prevented a number of physicians from employing it and underscored its unethical commercial features. At a medical society meeting in late 1885 in Washington, D.C., a physician reporting on the excellence of Antipyrine as a febrifuge could not remember the formula, which provoked another doctor to decry "the use of a drug of which we do not know the chemical constituents."[52] Although the comments of the other doctors at this meeting imply that they were suspicious of this medication and were treating it to some extent as a nostrum, this attitude was the minority opinion. The drug became popular and respected despite its commercialisms; it was simply too useful to ignore.

As for acetanilid, the inaugural German article in 1886 only used that word once or twice, introducing the discovery as Antifebrin, a term like Antipyrine that was obviously meant to suggest medical uses and which provoked criticism for that reason. (It also appeared in some journals as "antifibrin," a mistake the *American Druggist* found irritating.)[53] Antifebrin was, of course, the trade name registered to Kalle and Company, but it is clear that in the United States it was seen as the drug's "more convenient name," not as property (although several authors exhorted their readers to use the scientific term instead).[54] In Antifebrin's case at least, proper nomenclature was manageable, and "acetanilid" did appear quite frequently in the literature and occasionally in prescriptions.[55]

Bayer's product, on the other hand, first appeared in the medical literature as acetphenetidin and only some months later as Phenacetin. Furthermore, in the U.S. patent document, the only name provided for the "New Pharmaceutical Product" being described was Phenacetin—implying that this word was available for use by the public.[56] This might suggest that Bayer was behaving in a more professional manner by providing a convenient synonym and avoiding the improprieties of its competitors. But as we shall see in a later chapter, Bayer was in fact far more aggressive about its property rights than were either of the other German firms. And in any case, for the seventeen years of the patent it did not matter which of the two drugs American doctors prescribed—acetphenetidin or Phenacetin; every prescription in the United States was supposed to be filled with the Bayer product because Bayer was the only legal source of the drug.

Prescription records and publications alike suggest that from the start, American physicians were disinclined to use the scientific names when discussing or prescribing any of the German synthetic drugs.[57] Their habit of referring to them by their brand names annoyed the medical elite because it simply continued the bad practices associated with nostrum use—ignorance of ingredients, laziness, nonindividualized medical care, and other unprofessional habits. But there was another troubling aspect to the cavalier use of trade names: the opportunity for ordinary men and women to learn the name of the drug their doctors were ordering for them. Had antipyresis been the only therapeutic property these drugs possessed, it is very likely that they would have remained largely within the purview of the medical profession. Fevers were the sorts of ailments the public considered serious enough to seek a doctor's advice. But all three synthetics also demonstrated another, largely unanticipated, property: they were painkillers. And one of the pains they could kill was the headache.

An American doctor, John Blake White, was one of the first to discover that fifteen grains of Antipyrine given in a single dose "promptly relieves the symptom of headache whenever present, whether resulting from

disordered digestion, disturbances of the menstrual functions, loss of
sleep, undue mental effort, or even that associated with dreaded urae-
mia."[58] He also found that patients could take the drug prophylactically, to
ward off "recurrent attacks of cranial neuralgia." Another doctor reported
that in 1885 he had prescribed Antipyrine in eighteen cases of severe headache, migraine, or facial neuralgia, with only one failure. Four patients
with migraine, for example, told him the drug "acted like magic" and that
they had "never had anything so good." He also described five earlier cases
of severe headaches in which morphine and other remedies had been of
no avail and was convinced that in all these cases, "antipyrin would have
saved my patients much mental worry, and often the keenest physical suffering."[59] A Rhode island physician reported that "if antipyrine [was] not a
specific in certain forms of cephalalgia it certainly [came] nearer to it than
any preparation with which I have experimented." Treating his own headache, he had found that "almost immediately" after ten grains "the paroxysm [was] lessened, and within an hour or two there [was] complete relief."
In addition, subsequent migraines were less frequent and less intense. His
patients had had similar experiences, although the drug was not remarkable, he said, in frontal or digestive headaches.[60] Another practitioner told
colleagues at a medical meeting that he had found Antipyrine excellent in
migraine but less useful in malarial or dyspeptic headaches; it was quite
ineffective in uremic headache. A member of his audience added his own
observation that a "gastric headache following a debauch was promptly
mitigated by one or two doses."[61]

A New York doctor wrote to the *Medical Record* that this new medicine
relieved any kind of hemicrania (migraine) better than anything else he
had tried. His migraine patients, especially the nervous businessmen and
the overworked housewives, expecting the usual twelve to eighteen hours
of agony, now found relief in an hour.[62] Another New York practitioner
pointed out that patients who had been inconvenienced by the soporific
actions of the opiates had no such side effects when they took Antipyrine.
Moreover, the synthetic rarely failed to relieve the pain. It was not
unpleasant to the taste and produced no gastric upset. It did not seem to
be habit forming. In more than eighty cases of migraine, this doctor had
had favorable results in fifty-four and acceptable results in fifteen.[63] At
least one headache patient reported to his physician that Antipyrine was a

good substitute for the morphine he had used on other occasions, although the doctor himself had not found the synthetic particularly good for extreme pain.[64]

In similar fashion, Antifebrin (acetanilid) quickly proved to assuage pain in many febrile and nonfebrile conditions; headaches of various types were relieved promptly. A German investigator who tried Antifebrin for his own migraines was delighted to report that the pain was usually gone in thirty minutes to an hour. It was better than anything else he had used and in his opinion was "absolutely without danger, besides being cheap and without taste."[65] A Pennsylvania physician stated that in a one-year study of five hundred cases of headache, he had found this drug "a most effectual analgesic," "the remedy, par excellence, for sick headache," "and that, when used with the precautions necessary in the use of all drugs, it [was] absolutely without danger."[66] In treating the nervous headache of "delicate females," a doctor from Illinois preferred Antifebrin to Antipyrine because Antipyrine depressed the heart too much.[67] Another practitioner was similarly pleased to report that even when "administered recklessly," Antifebrin had not been associated with any fatalities.[68]

On the whole, however, the medical profession was less enthusiastic about acetanilid than Antipyrine and thought Antipyrine was the better headache remedy.[69] By the time Phenacetin appeared, the novelty of the German drugs had worn off to some degree and doctors had learned what to expect. So, although introduced as a febrifuge, Phenacetin's painkilling properties were noted almost immediately, and it was found to be capable of promptly relieving sciatica, neuralgia, as well as rheumatic and other pains.[70] Headaches, of course, were quite prominent in these descriptions: eighteen of the twenty-five patients to whom a German doctor successfully gave analgesic Phenacetin had been suffering from headaches.[71]

With these three synthetics, none of which was advertised to the public, the organic chemical industry had in effect given physicians powerful therapeutic agents with remarkable analgesic properties unprecedented in medical history. So we might expect that insofar as the headache was concerned, American doctors struggling to find respect, status, and authority would seize upon these drugs as an opportunity to enhance their image as compassionate, competent, and modern. The synthetics gave headache sufferers a real reason to seek professional advice. At last the cries of "Cannot you do something for these frightful headaches?" could be answered in the affirmative.[72] The drugs did not provide relief in all cases, but for many moderate headaches and even for some migraines they worked rapidly in nontoxic doses, with sustained action. They did not befuddle the patient. They did not appear to be habit forming. Delivered from hours of discomfort and misery, grateful men and women would learn to trust physicians for all medical matters, and professionals, mastering the latest scientific knowledge, would be seen to be worthy of that trust. So it may be somewhat surprising that in spite of the enthusiastic reports about the synthetics as headache remedies without peer, many of those practitioners whom we might call headache experts did not always appreciate these new medicines or were very cautious about them, even dismissive.

For one thing, the synthetics were not as benign as the first articles and reports had made them seem. Side effects were a hazard with any drug, but these new medicines produced an array of unfamiliar reactions that made some practitioners unwilling to use them. Reports of circulatory collapse became more common and alarming; the drugs were sometimes accused of being fatally poisonous even in small doses.[73] Some physicians also claimed that the painkillers were nearly as habit forming as the opiates and created equally depraved addicts.[74] Furthermore, the enthusiasm in the medical press put some doctors in mind of the worst proprietaries, so they took the claims for the drugs with a grain of salt. But the greatest misgivings about the German synthetics stemmed from the pervasive reluctance to accept painkilling as an appropriate medical goal, especially for an ailment with such myriad causes and manifestations as the headache. Despite the progress in pharmacology and related sciences, despite the growing acceptance of other kinds of symptomatic or specific treatments, the painkillers themselves had not advanced medical knowledge. They had done nothing to reveal the true causes of headaches. The drugs alleviated too many different kinds of headaches to be thought of as eradicating or affecting root causes. They were merely analgesics. Their use as such remained unacceptably empirical because they masked the best clue to the cause of the ailment. In headaches, causes remained the real target of treatment and the goal to which true professional practitioners should always aspire.[75] Besides, headaches were still often seen as a kind of retribution, the body's revenge for the abuses heaped upon it by men and women living hectic modern lives. Painkillers were an easy way out, an unrealistic attempt to avoid the pain that was the common lot of humanity.[76]

To a large extent, after a brief period of euphoria at the prospect of a pain panacea, cooler heads prevailed and reminded physicians of the dangers of this kind of empiricism. Unfortunately, advances in medical science had not revealed much about the pathology of headaches, and doctors were as much in darkness as ever. Some physicians continued to discuss the ailment in terms of temperament and disequilibrium, with multiple potential causes and possible remedies. As late as 1892 a New York doctor was describing patients' constitutions as sanguine or phlegmatic and classifying their headaches accordingly.[77] A doctor in Buffalo advised an old-fashioned tonic of nux vomica, gentian, phosphoric acid, and pepsin for congestive headaches resulting from prolonged brain work, along with sponge baths of cold salt water. ("If the heart is flagging, give a little digitalis.")[78] Such tonics could help "firm up" a system falling prey to the indolence of modern life. Eyestrain and nasal problems remained favorite culprits, in which case drug treatment provided "little or no benefit." Glasses were the "only permanent relief from headaches due to errors of refraction." For headaches of nasal origin, "mechanical and surgical measures judiciously selected for each case are much more to the purpose."[79] Laxatives were as popular as ever, especially in cases of toxemic headaches caused by autointoxication.[80]

Although after 1890 most discussions of the headache at least mentioned the new drugs, traditional nonanalgesic approaches were preferentially recommended. One advice book listed 96 different prescriptions plus 119 individual items that could be used alone or in combination. The list included the synthetics, but they were not given pride of place and appeared alongside leeches, baths, bleeding, and blisters.[81] Even as late as 1916, doctors could propose a visit to the seashore or the mountains, or massage, restriction of sexual activity, or a long stay at a sanatorium, depending on the particulars of the diagnosis and on the characteristics of the patient. Painkillers could be given if the pain was "unusually severe," but this clearly was not meant to be the final goal of treatment.[82]

Not all American practitioners were so reluctant to address the issue of headache pain, and they chided their colleagues for being "too prone to accept it as a necessary evil." The coal tar products could provide "immediate relief," although "they should be given with discretion; opiates very seldom if ever, better almost never."[83] As Buffalo, New York, practitioner Floyd Crego noted, pain had "no degree by which it [could] be gauged." Only the patient knew how much he or she was suffering. It was fortunate, he thought, that "to break up the attacks, we possess at present very useful remedies—namely, antipyrin, antifebrin, phenacetin and exalgyn [sic]."[84] Yet Crego's choice of words is instructive because it suggests that he viewed the drugs not so much as masking the pain but as somehow neutralizing the nerve "attack" that caused the pain—a more permissible rationale for their use. This is similar to nineteenth-century descriptions of quinine as interrupting a malarial paroxysm to abort the fever. Because "official" headache treatment still promoted the laxatives, emetics and soporifics that were thought to correct, obstruct, or otherwise interfere with the cause of the ache, the synthetics were more acceptable when prescribed for their presumed sedative rather than for their known pain-killing, effects.

Even so, such endorsements of analgesia as a reasonable first resort were rare, although the constant reminders in the medical journals to seek causes is perhaps evidence that many physicians in fact prescribed the new painkillers far more often than they admitted, simply because it was expedient. But, as Daniel Clark of Toronto admitted, although pain relief was desirable and the "much-lauded" synthetic palliatives might "comfortably tide over an attack," the next and more important step was "to cure, if possible, the disease by using remedies which tend to bring about a better condition in the system."[85] Whatever else they might do, analgesics were usually not thought to work in that way. Dealing with headache therefore remained "one of the most complex questions of therapeutics" that doctors faced, calling on all their skills as diagnosticians and prescribers. It was important that each patient learn *not* to expect immediate relief, so that the physician could establish a "rational hygienic and therapeutic course best adapted to the case."[86] Treating symptoms alone was simply not good medicine, no matter how grateful the patient. The diagnosis always took precedence.[87] It was very unfortunate that the most important symptom was also the most unpleasant, but after all, "Pain was the price of life."[88] Patients, however, did not necessarily agree.

Having initially been prescribed Antipyrine, Phenacetin, or Antifebrin for their fevers or influenza, the American public soon realized that of all the symptoms they suffered, their headaches and other pains were the ones these drugs relieved most agreeably and most quickly. It was from patients' reports, after all, that the medical world had first learned of this property. It also did not take the public long to realize that even if physicians were reluctant to order the drugs as painkillers, people could always prescribe for themselves. Anyone could purchase these drugs from any pharmacy simply by asking for them. Although ethical, the synthetics were not restricted, and the same features that made the synthetics popular with the medical profession made them accessible to the laity: easily remembered names and the fact that no other ingredients were necessary in the recipe. One word alone was sufficient to obtain efficacious treatment. These drugs, complained one commentator in 1889, "have already passed the stage where the trade is confined to prescriptions. The druggists now sell them over the counter in bulk as they do the cinchona alkaloids." The synthetics, he predicted, would rival anything that had come before them.[89] Prophetic words indeed.

5

Druggists, Doctors, and the Law

Whether nostrums or ethicals, German or American, professionally prescribed or self-administered, virtually all drugs by the last quarter of the
nineteenth century reached the public by way of a pharmacy. Although
pharmacists are often overlooked by historians, they nevertheless had an
important role in a culture in which both lay and professional practices
relied so heavily on drugs and in which jurisdictional boundaries were not
always well defined. Some of the same issues that plagued American
doctors in their efforts to establish themselves as professionals also con-
fronted pharmacists, but—unlike doctors, who eventually achieved a powerful position in American society and became models of a professional
elite—druggists became primarily shopkeepers. They were respectable
enough but tainted to some extent by commerce. American pharmacists,
in fact, labored under two perennial difficulties. One was the problem of
reconciling their scientific and professional objectives with their business
interests. The other was their subordination to physicians whose knowledge of pharmaceutical chemistry was often less than that of the druggists.
Throughout the nineteenth century there was a core of reformers who
worked diligently to establish high standards of practice, but by the last
two decades of the century, circumstances conspired to make some of
these professional goals irrelevant. The headache remedies are a particularly good example of the problems pharmacists faced in the nineteenth
and early twentieth centuries, revealing the tensions that existed between
pharmacists and doctors, the stresses imposed by the increasingly com-

mercial aspects of pharmaceutical supply, and the implications these had for the public.

In the colonial and early republican eras, the difference between pre-scribers and dispensers (and laymen) was often moot: Benjamin Franklin, for example, "dabbled in both professions without being educated in either."[1] Although there were a few individuals who specialized in phar-macy, for the most part the physician-apothecary remained the norm well into the nineteenth century. By the 1820s, however, influenced by the chemical revolution in France and Germany, American pharmaceutical practitioners had begun to establish themselves as distinct from physi-cians, claiming as their domain all those matters pertaining to the identi-fication and preparation of medicinal products.

Compounding a prescription was no mere handicraft. A pharmacist had to know the medicinal, chemical, toxic, and physical properties of whatever he was called upon to dispense. He was expected to transform leaves, barks, and roots into powders, solutions, tinctures, or elixirs. He had to mix stubborn and uncooperative ingredients into gummy masses, rolling out the pills by hand, hoping that each pill contained more or less the same amount of active ingredient. Too little, and there would be no effect; too much, and he might kill the patient. He worked with noxious, often dangerous chemicals such as arsenic and cyanide, and volatile and explosive ones such as ether. Like the doctor, he was on call night and day. But unlike the doctor, he rarely got any credit. The success of a prescrip-tion would always be assigned to the physician; its failure might well be blamed on the druggist.

By midcentury, pharmacists generally agreed that their skills and knowledge did not authorize them to diagnose or prescribe in the same manner as physicians, but they did think they were entitled to be consid-ered doctors' colleagues. It was druggists, after all, who guaranteed that the physician's (supposedly) carefully considered and complicated prescription was dispensed correctly. It was a point of professional pride for a druggist to declare that in his shop, "no medicines [would] be put up unless of the first quality."[2] Quality ingredients, of course, guarded against the adulteration that was the cause of "much of the uncertainty attendant upon the admin-istration of medicines."[3] The need to accurately identify impurities and adulterants was one of the major justifications for the existence of an organized, self-policing pharmaceutical profession, which began to take shape in the 1820s with the founding of the first schools and associations, and the first edition of the *United States Pharmacopoeia* (*USP*).[4] It was not until the American Pharmaceutical Association (APhA) was established in 1852, however, that a real profession of pharmacy can be said to have existed in the United States.[5] Like the AMA, the APhA established criteria for membership, defined the boundaries of professional practice, agitated for improved education, campaigned for better licensing laws, and formulated a code of ethics that, among other things, insisted that members "uphold the use of the [United States] Pharmacopoeia in their practice."[6]

In creating the *USP*, its compilers had intended to set out national standards of strength, purity, and nomenclature for the items in practice. Earlier versions of pharmacopeias, either European or American, had tended to be lists of items commonly used, often with sample prescriptions and prescribing advice. They were often not much different from botanical handbooks with recipes, instructing the reader how to identify medicinal substances and prepare various remedies. Hence they were as popular with the laity as with apothecaries. The *USP*, on the other hand, a deliberate attempt to establish truly professional, scientific criteria for medicinal substances, was too technical for the average member of the public.[7] (For the most part, it considered only single entities and compounds rather than combinations. Guidelines for formulas were not published until the APhA compiled the first *National Formulary* in 1888.) Revised every ten years, the *USP* neither condemned nor endorsed any particular drug. It reflected, rather than guided, contemporary practice, leaving the choice of approved items to the medical profession. Technical matters were left to pharmacists. Nevertheless it was especially uncompromising in its efforts to establish a scientific foundation for American materia medica. As a result, the *USP* was adamant that such egregious commercialisms as trade names and patents should immediately disqualify an item from inclusion. For the first seventy years of its existence, this was not a difficult standard to maintain: no legitimate drug had a patent, and every item in use had a well-known common or Latin name.[8] Pharmacists who dispensed only *USP* items were therefore in no danger of violating another provision of the code, which required them to discontinue the use of secret formulas and "to discountenance quackery and dishonorable competition in their business." Even before the creation of the APhA, many American druggists had been offended by the proliferation of nostrums and had proudly proclaimed that such "patent medicines [were] not manufactured or sold" at their establishments.[9] The APhA was simply echoing an already widely held view of what a professional druggist was supposed to be.

The APhA code also did not allow members to counterprescribe, that is, to supply a remedy for a customer who was actually asking for medical advice. Proprietaries, of course, made counterprescribing all the easier, as did the public's long-standing habit of asking druggists for suggestions and recommendations. But if pharmacists were to earn doctors' respect (and their prescription business), they had to leave all prescribing to the medical profession. (In recognition of the realities of the American situation, the code in fact only stipulated that pharmacists should avoid prescribing "when practicable" and did not forbid the practice outright, but it nevertheless remained the ideal.) In return, however, physicians, were supposed to honor their pharmaceutical brethren by refraining from doing their own dispensing and by writing accurate, intelligent prescriptions that would require some skill and ingenuity to prepare. Thus druggists found it especially disheartening that in spite of their own efforts to become more professional as dispensers, many doctors were becoming even fonder of proprietaries and other readymade concoctions, a tendency that accelerated after the Civil War.

In a three-month period in 1889, Mahlon N. Kline of the Philadelphia jobbing concern of Smith and Kline Company examined the orders sent to his firm from five leading pharmacies in five eastern cities. On average, 59 percent of every order was for patent medicines and proprietaries. Of 1,125 orders sent in from March through May, only two did not request proprietary articles. Kline acknowledged that the druggists could have purchased *USP* items from another wholesaler, but four of the five stores, he said, used Smith and Kline almost exclusively for all their needs, and four also had large prescription businesses. Clearly, these pharmacies were dispensing many prescriptions with branded products.[10] A survey in 1895 found that 27.4 percent of prescriptions contained a proprietary of some sort, including such things as Vaseline and Listerine.[11] According to one critic there were 36,500 unoriginal mixtures in existence in the United States, each known "by some particular name," all of them "totally unworthy." Their use in prescriptions, he said, was demoralizing to the pharmaceutical profession.[12] Nor was it just the average physician who was guilty of these practices. One druggist said he had received prescriptions "ordering not only proprietary but really patent medicines . . . [from] men who [occupied] leading positions among their brethren."[13]

Even when doctors did attempt to prescribe extemporaneously, said their critics, they were putting patients in harm's way by being "ignorant of certain facts in chemistry, which every apothecary knows by rote."[14] Druggists' periodicals made frequent, often sarcastic references to illegible, illiterate, ridiculous, or dangerous prescriptions their local doctors wanted filled, with "bad spelling, bad Latin, contractions, bad writing, unofficinal names, terms of doubtful meaning," and other offenses, but these at least posed a challenge of sorts to the dispenser.[15] The proprietary order did not. "What encouragement is there to pharmacists to become skillful and experts," asked one sympathetic medical man, "if the physicians of their vicinity make no demand upon them for skill and knowledge?"[16] "Because a few proprietary articles possess merit and have found favor with the practitioner, a thousand imitations under new names, and in gaudy dress, have made, and continue to make their appearance until it is absolutely nauseating."[17] A physician who used a pre-made formula was "little better than an empiric."[18] As one druggist noted wryly, "The great number of proprietary mixtures advertised and sampled to physicians as symptomatic cures, must make it indeed very easy to practice medicine."[19]

In fact, practicing medicine had become so easy that doctors were even teaching their patients to do it, according to the *New York Times*:

> [A physician] writes out a prescription for a standard preparation and gives it to a patient. The patient is one of the knowing kind, like the majority of patients, and when he reads the name of some well-known patent medicine man on his prescription he immediately resolves to outwit the physician. Going to the apothecary shop, he says to the clerk, "Give me a bottle of Blank's uh-uh-ah-ah, lemme see." He has forgotten what Blank's remedy is called, and he tugs at the prescription in his pocket and reads it. "Oh yes," he resumes, "give me a bottle of Blank's High-and-Mighty Bazouk."[20]

By using the brand name, the doctor had given the patient unlimited access to a powerful medicine as well as to information (listed on the label of Blank's Bazouk) about other diseases or symptoms for which that medicine claimed some effectiveness and from which the patient might now be convinced he suffered. Having lost confidence in the doctor, he would diagnose and treat himself, his family, and his friends (and save himself a fee into the bargain).[21] It was up to the doctors themselves, however, to prevent this scenario. Pharmacists could help by encouraging doctors "not to be bulldozed by the large manufacturers," but physicians must learn to prescribe by individual, pharmacopeial items.[22] The trouble was, doctors did not seem inclined to take this advice.

Despite the AMA's admittedly modest efforts late in the century to inculcate pharmacopeial prescribing habits, many American practitioners were simply not willing to abandon proprietaries and were not necessarily sympathetic to the pharmacists' point of view.[23] Moreover, pharmacists were required by protocol, if not by law, to dispense *exactly* what the doctor requested (unless it was a dangerous error) and were liable to prosecution for any mistakes—a strong incentive to provide good service and to not countermand doctors. Yet some doctors said they ordered proprietaries because they did not have confidence in druggists: they suspected pharmacists of dispensing inferior materials.[24] Other doctors accused druggists of making unauthorized substitutions in prescriptions or taking kickbacks from manufacturers.[25] Dispensing errors were thought to be common. The *New York Tribune*, for example, reported that drugstore clerks, who worked long hours with little social life, were easily distracted by chatting while on duty and therefore mixed the wrong ingredients.[26] There was some foundation for all these criticisms. The demands for better pharmaceutical education, like the demands for better medical education, had not yet resulted in uniformly trained pharmacists. Many states did not even require high school graduation before entrance to a pharmacy program, and it was not until 1932 that a man or woman needed a bachelor of science degree in pharmacy in order to dispense medications.[27]

In the meantime, the two professions continued to bicker. The prescription itself became a bone of contention. Who, in fact, owned it—the doctor, the druggist, or the patient? Could a pharmacist legitimately refill one without the physician's approval? Some druggists did not hesitate to do so, even though this could easily be interpreted as counterprescribing. In fact, one New York medical association accused the APhA of equivocating on this question for pecuniary reasons and demanded that unauthorized renewals be made a misdemeanor, although the physicians failed to obtain the necessary legislation. For its part, the APhA maintained that it was simply not possible to prevent refills.[28] Other solutions that physicians suggested were to boycott offending druggists or to dispense from the doctor's office.[29] As one practitioner noted, the pharmaceutical industry's prepared drugs were now so convenient that physicians did not need to use druggists at all. They could even take their medicines along on house calls.[30] Pharmacists, for their part, accused doctors who dispensed their own medicines of being either selfish or ignorant, but with so many elegant proprietaries available, druggists were afraid that if the number of dispensing physicians became large enough, pharmacists' business would indeed suffer.[31]

American pharmacists, in fact, could not make a living on their prescription trade alone. In Europe, regulations restricted the number of apothecaries in any given location and allowed them to concentrate on the scientific aspects of their vocation, but in America, the drug and drugstore business became very commercial and competitive very early: by 1851 in Baltimore alone there were already about one hundred apothecary shops.[32] Stores had to develop other ways to attract customers and quickly departed from strictly pharmaceutical pursuits. It was appropriate for druggists to create or at least to sell tooth powders, rat poisons, insect powders, perfumes, cosmetics, soaps, and other similar commodities that called upon their expertise in chemistry. By allowing these products in their shops, pharmacists in theory could guarantee their quality and maintain professional supervision of goods that affected the public's health. At the same time, however, drugstores began to sell stationery, tobacco, notions, hair brushes, bath mats, and postage stamps. In the 1850s the soda fountain began to appear; an offshoot of the medicinal uses of "waters," it quickly became a refreshment emporium. By the 1880s many drugstores boasted elaborate ice cream parlors and lunch counters, and pharmaceutical journals featured hints about making cherry phosphates and ham sandwiches, along with the latest discoveries from Europe and information about detecting adulterants in medicines. Retailing techniques were becoming as crucial as pharmaceutical knowledge.

Some of the most lucrative commodities druggists sold were the very items against which both professional pharmacy and medicine competed—the "public" nostrums. The patent medicines that were lavishly advertised in the newspapers and magazines of the nation were in fact essential for the survival of many shops. They drew a steady clientele to the store with little risk or bother to the owner, even though profit margins were low. Although reform-minded pharmacists despised patent medicines, failure to stock them simply meant that the customers went elsewhere. Keeping the items in stock might also mean having to "sell" them, a job so distasteful to one high-minded drugstore clerk that he refused to recommend *any* patent medicine, although if the customer insisted on buying it, he would sell it. (When the manufacturers heard about this, they wanted his employer to dismiss him.)[33] Nostrums were so popular and so ubiquitous, in fact, that the ethical ban on them was impossible to maintain. As early as 1855 the APhA dropped adherence to this clause in its code of ethics as a requirement for membership, recognizing that to stay in business a pharmacist had no choice but to deal in these kinds of items.

Despite these drawbacks, however, pharmacy was an attractive occupation. Between 1820 and 1880, nineteen professional schools were established; by 1900 there were forty-five more.[34] By the turn of the century, more than 57,000 men and women were in the retail drug business in the United States.[35] Even without a huge prescription business, a drugstore could provide a decent living. In 1857, the owner of the Limerick Drug Store in Rodney, Mississippi, claimed he did between $10,000 and $12,000 worth of business annually.[36] He was trying to sell the store, so his figures may have been a little inflated, but thirty years later the manufacturing pharmacist Edward Squibb calculated that "a moderate dispensing store" could clear $1,800 a year in profits.[37]

According to the *Therapeutic Gazette* in 1882, drugstores were more in demand than doctors because they provided what people wanted (or what the advertising had convinced them they wanted).[38] This demand did not make use of the pharmacist's professional skills, but an enterprising man could nevertheless turn it to his advantage by distracting customers from the brand-name article and selling them the druggist's own house version or private brand instead. These were cheaper than the nationally advertised brands, with the added benefit of being professionally (and personally) formulated and supervised. Such activities could very well enhance the pharmacist's reputation in the neighborhood, but doctors often suspected that it was at the medical profession's expense. One Hoboken physician conjectured that his local druggists' friendly habit of welcoming new physicians was simply an attempt to persuade the doctors to send business their way. Once they acquired a prescription order, the druggists could then offer renewals without the patient's having to go back to the doctor. And they never sent their customers to seek medical advice if they could sell them something instead.[39]

Druggists, on the other hand, claimed that if doctors would just prescribe properly and professionally, pharmacists would have no need to resort to any kind of nostrums or any real counterprescribing. They would be happy to send doctors all the patients they could handle. At the same time, however, "the extreme view that no drug should be given except upon the advice of a physician cannot be maintained without carrying the argument to absurdity. For the exclusive right to prescribe carries with it the exclusive right to declare when a person needs prescriptions, and this demands a constant attendance upon the doctor that is preposterous."[40] There were many instances when a druggist was "called upon for a remedy for a cold, bilious attack, or similar light ailments, and it [was] perfectly proper for him to furnish such articles as may be suitable."[41]

Until the introduction of the German synthetics, however, headache was usually not listed as an appropriately light ailment (testimony once again to the difficulties it presented and to the equivocal status of "painkilling" in professional medical thinking). But with the arrival of Antipyrine and the other German drugs, the situation changed dramatically. The analgesic antipyretics are in fact good examples of how druggists facilitated the public's access to the sort of remedies that the medical elites, and some of the pharmaceutical elites, thought should be used only on the advice of a physician. It was also a situation that some members of the lay community began to comment on. The *New York Tribune*, for instance, noted that in Belgium not even quinine could be purchased without a prescription, but in New York City the synthetics were available just for the asking. And the principal reason people asked was because they had headaches.[42]

Records of the Niagara Apothecary in Ontario are tantalizingly suggestive of the popularity of headache powders in the 1890s. The day books list all sales the store made. Before the 1890s, there are a few references to "powders"—Seidlitz, tooth, face powder, and so on. In the 1890s, however, there are frequent (once or more a day) entries of "powder," sold for five cents. This was the usual price for five grains of acetanilid, and these entries very likely refer to headache remedies.[43] By the early 1890s, many drug journals had begun to supply formulas for various headache preparations, most based on acetanilid, which, at fifty cents a pound, could produce more than 1,100 five-grain powders for mere fractions of a cent.[44] Huge potential profits also attracted large-scale nostrum manufacturers, of course, and advertisements for Antidolorine, Mattern's Headache Powder, Antinervin, Mascot Headache Cure, Pyro-Febrin Tablets ("The Best Cure on Earth for Headaches"), Gessler's Magic Headache Wafers, Armstrong's Headache Powder (200 samples and three dozen twenty-five-cent-size packages, plus "plenty of booklets" titled "Facts, A Few on Headache," all for $5.00), and Antikamnia began to appear in the pharmaceutical press. Oddly, however, such advertisements did not appear in the lay press; nor did they appear in the medical press—less oddly, perhaps, given the medical profession's distaste for symptomatic treatments. In dental journals, for example, where we might expect pain to be an important topic, anesthesia was discussed (and anesthetics widely advertised), but postoperative dental pain received little mention, perhaps because it was so obviously a short-term experience, however much the patient might suffer for a few days.[45] As in medical journals, advertisements for analgesics are hard to find in dental literature.

Antikamnia was a significant exception to this general rule. A self-proclaimed ethical painkiller as well as a homegrown synthetic, it was widely and attractively advertised in nearly every medical and pharmaceutical periodical of the day (including *JAMA*) and is worth a second look because it was a prominent example of the kind of "ethical proprietary" that both the AMA and APhA found so troublesome. First marketed in 1890 by the Antikamnia Company of St. Louis as a proudly American but strictly ethical drug, Antikamnia was, at about one dollar per ounce,

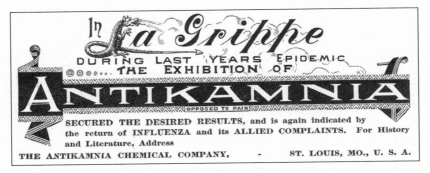

FIGURE 4. One of the multitudes of Antikamnia advertisements.
From *Pacific Drug Review* (1892).

competitive with Phenacetin and became very popular with physicians. It could also be obtained in various formulations (with quinine, with salol, later with heroin and other medicines), as a powder, or in tablets of one to ten grains. At no point did the Missouri manufacturer identify the product as anything other than Antikamnia, which implied that it was a chemical entity in the same way that Phenacetin or Antifebrin were.

Upon inspection, however, "several peculiarities . . . gave rise to the suspicion that a mere mixture of several compounds was under examination." Finding, in fact, that Antikamnia was nothing more than equal parts of acetanilid and bicarbonate of soda, with a little tartaric acid thrown in for good measure, one analyst pointed out that "the mixture [could] be prepared for about 10 cents per ounce, for which the manufacturers charge[d] $1.10."[46] Another analyst found that his sample contained about 78 percent acetanilid, a little less than 20 percent sodium bicarbonate, the remainder being "impurities."[47] The St. Louis firm took umbrage at this and responded that, in the first place, all such analyses were basically incorrect, and in the second place, it was not just the proportion of ingredients that counted but the process of manufacture—a trade secret. Besides, to date the company had received 3,792 positive endorsements.[48] Antikamnia, in fact, was an outrageous example of a nostrum masquerading as a legitimate pharmaceutical (which made its manufacturers millionaires).[49] To medical reformers, however, its success was further evidence of the deficiencies of American practitioners and the allure of symptomatic remedies. Nevertheless, Antikamnia remained one of the few painkillers ever advertised as such.

Even in the drug journals, all of which carried advertisements for patent medicines as well as ethicals, copy for headache remedies is surprisingly less prevalent than that for diet supplements, tonics, and other popular nostrums. According to the critics of patent remedies, the most exuberant promotion of painkillers took place in the nation's magazines and newspapers, but even here one is far less likely to come across a headache cure than cures for "male weakness" (impotence), "female irregularities" (pregnancy), and, of course, the "saved-from-the-brink-of-death" miracle cures available from any drugstore or by mail. It was not a matter of taste or decorum, then, that kept headache powders out of papers like the *Washington Post* or the *New York Tribune*. The *Tribune*, in fact, devoted an entire page to Swift's Sure Specific in 1886 (18 July). Headache powder advertisements, however, are exceedingly scarce and are rarely found even in small-town papers. Anecdotal evidence suggests that church papers and other unsophisticated publications were a prime location for painkiller advertising, but in fact it may have been drugstore windows that helped make the headache powder a fact of American life at the turn of the century.[50]

By the mid-1890s, pharmaceutical journals had begun to provide frequent instructions on how to set up inviting window and counter displays to entice headache remedy purchasers.[51] Jobbing printers happily supplied large quantities of attractive cartons, labels, pill boxes, and bottles, custom designed or already stamped "Headache Powder." Drug journals such as the *Therapeutic Gazette* thought it "highly advisable . . . that [pharmacists] prepare their own powders, know exactly how much of each ingredient they contain, and fortify them (if necessary) with cardiac stimulants."[52] (In fact, a Pennsylvania retail druggists' association decided to stamp the packages of a particular headache nostrum as "contents unknown," which prompted the manufacturer to threaten them with a law suit for mutilating the packages.)[53] It was better for pharmacists to make their own headache remedies because it gave them an opportunity to demonstrate their skills and provided a humane service for their customers; it also allowed them to guarantee the final product. By creating house brands, pharmacists restored a professional, scientific component to their activities. Furthermore, all headache powders appear to have been promoted and sold in small quantities and were not intended to be kept on hand in the family medicine chest. This meant that headache sufferers had to come to the druggist every time they needed relief, and in a sense their use of these drugs could be supervised.

By the turn of the century the headache powder had become a well-established article of commerce, very popular with the public, and available as national or private brands in any pharmacy. Chronic sufferers and patients with severe headaches might continue to consult physicians, but the occasional or "garden-variety" pain could be readily relieved by a visit to the local druggist. Certainly the quantities being sold strongly suggest that most Americans believed the powders would be effective. Doctors protested this cavalier attitude to a symptom they still considered to be an important diagnostic sign, but their complaints usually stayed within the profession. As a group, they were still too ineffective to influence legislation, public opinion, or the behavior of pharmacists. And given the behavior of physicians, pharmacists saw no good reason to stop selling powders to the public. It was one way to compensate for the loss of their traditional responsibilities, substantially eroded by the modern drug industry and incompetent practitioners. (Besides, druggists could do no more harm to patients than, for instance, the practitioner who prescribed "as much as 60 grains of acetphenetidine daily . . . as 'palliative' treatment for headache.")[54] Pharmacists could analyze commercial powders and concoct better versions themselves. They were better equipped, they thought, to be the de facto managers of the drugs the public demanded for the self-treatment of headache. It was apparently a profitable situation—the powders did a steady business. But this very popularity was itself increasingly problematic. Druggists could not in fact monitor self-medication any more than doctors could. Within about ten years, it was claimed that "no class of remedies [was] subject to more abuse than the so-called headache cures."[55] It would not be the medical profession, however, that took the first steps to deal with this problem.

Preoccupied with getting its own house in order, more concerned about the companies that traded "on the innocent credulity of the regular physician" than those that preyed on the public, and trying to determine how best to keep physicians from prescribing proprietaries (one suggestion was to shame these doctors publicly), the AMA at the turn of the century was neither prepared nor inclined to address the question of limiting public access to drugs.[56] Reform-minded doctors in general deplored the public's use of nostrums as dangerous and railed at the druggists for aiding and abetting, but outside the editorial pages they made no obvious effort to ban, control, or otherwise regulate these products. The AMA apparently hoped that as regular practitioners became more professional and therefore more attractive, patients would learn to trust their physicians and reject the nostrums. What actions the AMA took on the question of proprietaries were for the most part directed to producing this trustworthy, educated doctor.

Even so, the AMA's efforts to encourage scientific prescribing appear to have been halfhearted. It was not until April 1900 that *JAMA* began a series of articles "designed to correct the abuses of advertising and patronizing pharmaceutical specialties."[57] It was short-lived, however. Eight essays had appeared by mid-July but no more, "and the work . . . was left incomplete without any explanation."[58] Although *JAMA* did refuse to advertise certain preparations and claimed to have already lost $8,000 in revenue on this account, the association "failed to live up to its pledge of purging its own publication of unfit advertisements."[59] Unable to influence even its own members, the AMA certainly had no voice that lawmakers cared to listen to. Nostrums continued to flourish.

Americans who now found the drug situation intolerable were unwilling to wait for doctors to take the initiative. Appalled by the growing number of stories about patent medicines that turned men, women, and children into dope fiends, and mothers and infants into drunks, temperance advocates, health reformers, and various do-gooders finally took the matter in hand around the turn of the century. Progressivism (the latest manifestation of the periodic American urge to improve the nation and its inhabitants), coupled with rise of consumer activism, had already primed the country for widespread reforms, addressing political corruption and other scandals, as well as social issues, by using the mass media of the day to convey its message. Large-circulation newspapers and magazines, many with national readerships, thus became powerful instruments of change. According to historian Richard Hofstadter, "To an extraordinary degree the work of the Progressive movement rested upon its journalism."[60] Conspicuous among the media were the muckrakers, whose shocking exposés of sweatshops, prisons, and other horrors seized the public's attention,

eliciting sympathy for society's unfortunate victims. But when the muckrakers turned to matters that affected middle-class readers personally—the
filthy state of food processing and the poisonous contents of patent medicines—the public became angry and aroused, demanding legislation to
protect American consumers.[61] For the food industry it was a piece of fiction—Upton Sinclair's 1906 novel *The Jungle*—that provoked a great outcry.
For the nostrum trade it was the series of articles on the Patent Medicine
Curse that appeared in *Ladies' Home Journal* and *Collier's Weekly* between
May 1904 and September 1906 that convinced the American middle class
it was being poisoned.

Samuel Hopkins Adams's articles in *Collier's* were particularly scathing.
He was not reluctant to name names and included illustrations of the
packages as well, so there would be no doubt as to the identity of the
offending item.[62] Virtually all patent medicines, Adams said, were frauds,
even those with some intrinsic value such as Pond's Extract (witch hazel).
Unfortunately, the manufacturer in this case did not restrict its advertising
"to decent methods, but in the recent epidemic scare in New York it traded
on the public alarm by putting forth 'display' advertisements headed, in
heavy black type, 'Meningitis,' a disease in which witch-hazel is about as
effective as molasses."[63] Even more dangerous, of course, were the concoctions that allowed men, women, and children to ingest some of the most
potent poisons known, especially alcohol, cocaine, and the opiates.

Adams also had a special place for the headache cures:

> Acetanilid will undoubtedly relieve headache of certain kinds; but
> acetanilid, as the basis of headache powders, is prone to remove the
> cause of the symptoms permanently by putting a complete stop to
> the heart action. Invariably, when taken steadily, it produces con-
> stitutional disturbances of insidious development which result
> fatally if the drug be not discontinued, and often it enslaves the
> devotee to its use.

In "The Subtle Poisons" (2 December 1905) Adams listed twenty-two Americans alleged to have died because they took acetanilid in headache remedies or bracers. ("This list does not include the case of a dog in Altoona,
Pa., which died immediately on eating some sample headache powders.
The dog did not know any better.") Not only sudden death awaited the

unsuspecting. "Patient use of these drugs will even produce an interesting and picturesque, if not intrinsically beautiful, purplish-gray hue of the face and neck." Addiction, too, could result, said Adams, with all the depravity and deceit associated with that affliction.[64] Adams did not find acetanilid itself to be unworthy but recommended its use only on the advice of a physician and excoriated the headache remedy industry for its failure to identify the contents of its products. He was particularly contemptuous of the industry's claims that it marketed only harmless ingredients.

The series in the *Ladies' Home Journal* (from which patent medicine advertising had been banned early on), written by editor Edward Bok, appealed to the maternal instincts of its readers, shocking them with revelations that the alcohol content of some favorite nostrums was greater than that of straight whisky and that by giving such remedies to their children or taking them during pregnancy, American mothers were creating a generation of drunkards and drug addicts. In fact, the *Journal* seems to have been upset less by the prospect of being poisoned than by the revelation that the patent medicine companies were selling each other the confidential and sometimes heart-rending letters women sent them, seeking advice about their own and their families' ailments.[65] (Bok was a well-known opponent of suffrage, working women—although his magazine advertised nursing schools—and female emancipation. He supported a genteel, domestic vision of American womanhood.)[66]

One article in the series was devoted to the headache powders, calling acetanilid "so dangerous that even the most skillful physicians nowadays are refusing to prescribe it."[67] Although it was known that women were far more likely than men to use these preparations, the *Journal* did not dwell on the powders and did not identify any brands by name. Readers were simply advised to avoid the whole class of remedies and consult their physicians rather than treat themselves. At the same time, however, Bok conceded that only in an ideal world would the habit of self-drugging disappear.[68] He therefore added the *Journal*'s voice to the growing clamor for an effective federal law, which would offer some protection to consumers.

Bok also seems to have had a more idealistic view of doctors than the doctors perhaps deserved at this point. Although it was true that medical use of acetanilid had fallen off in the first few years of the new century, it is not clear that this was because of the drug's purported dangers. Many doctors had used it as an antipyretic and now simply preferred Phenacetin for that purpose. A Philadelphia doctor complained that the drug was still prescribed so much it could result in a "disastrous association with other remedies."[69] Still, there was an increase in the number of demands from physicians that it not be used for self-treatment and in the number of published reports of its hazards: chronic poisoning (and slow decline), acute poisoning (and sudden death, even after just one dose),[70] and damage to the heart. A Kansas doctor was of the opinion that since the 1890 census (the first following the introduction of the coal tar drugs), deaths from heart disease had risen dramatically because of acetanilid use.[71] Similarly, *JAMA* thought that headache powders were to blame for the prevalence of "weak hearts and weak general circulation" that compromised the contemporary medical treatment "of all acute disease or post-operative conditions."[72] Nonetheless, these reports appear to have been a reaction to the muckraking campaign rather than the inspiration for it. Overall, in fact, there was a "relative lack of interest on the part of physicians" in the crusade against nostrums.[73] Although *JAMA* approved of the muckrakers and encouraged its readers to do battle with the patent medicine interests, it paid only lip service to the campaign in 1904.[74]

The next year, *JAMA* again praised Bok for advocating that no drug be used without a doctor's supervision and for his "strong and convincing plea for the exercise of ordinary good judgement before succumbing to the almost universal passion for self-medication" fostered by newspaper advertising.[75] Other professional journals were similarly opposed to the "great nostrum evil" but thought it would be difficult to deal with the problem of self-medication because "most laymen are thoroughly convinced that no matter what sickness befalls them, there is some drug which will help or cure them. It is practically impossible for many a patient to be treated without medicine, and if it is not given he will buy nostrums advertised by the lay press or by almanacs."[76] Indeed, doctors might have felt a twinge of guilt, because "So long as we cling to the habit of prescribing something, whether the patient needs it or not . . . so long are we encouraging the delusion that the real value of the physician lies in the drugs that he gives." Patients self-medicated on the same principle.[77]

The medical profession, in other words, had its own inadequacies to overcome before it could become an unequivocal supporter of the antinostrum campaign. The Pure Food and Drug Act passed in 1906 really owed its existence to Harvey W. Wiley, chief chemist in the Department of Agriculture, whose primary concern was *food* adulteration. He was a late-comer to the campaign against nostrums, although once they were in his sights he targeted them just as energetically as he targeted alum-laced flour or rat parts in sausages. But on the whole, the effort to warn the public about the dangers of proprietary drugs was initiated by laymen.[78] Nevertheless, this fact did no harm to doctors, about whom both Bok and Adams were flatteringly clear: they flatly told readers to consult their physicians before taking any medicine at all (and certainly before dosing their children).

Such support for doctors was fortuitous for the AMA. Disorganized, ineffective, and perceived as elitist, the AMA by 1900 had managed to entice less than 10 percent of the country's regular doctors to become members.[79] Concerned with its own shortcomings, the association had in fact undertaken a major reorganization in 1901 and seems to have been caught somewhat off guard by the muckrakers' crusades, which could account for its tepid response to them. But now that public opinion of patent medicines was so incensed by the exposés, the AMA's members "saw the advantages to professionalization of being linked with progressive reforms."[80] Supporting a movement designed for the public's benefit presented the AMA in a good light and fit very well into its plans to reform education and practice standards. With the abominations of Lydia Pinkham's Vegetable Compound and Pe-ru-na revealed to the average American, how could a self-respecting medical professional continue to prescribe their "ethical" equivalents? Thus *JAMA*, beginning in earnest in 1905, revived the commentaries on commercial drugs left dormant a few years earlier and published dozens of editorials, letters, and articles denouncing the nostrum evil.[81] These commentaries urged doctors to learn the art of scientific prescribing, in Latin, by reading the *USP* or other respectable volume, arguing that even so little as half an hour a week devoted to this task would "familiarize the physician with many a good medicament and teach him its composition."[82]

The AMA did more than write editorials this time, however. To ensure that its contempt for nostrums was based on scientific facts and as part of its efforts to improve education, in early 1905 it established a Council on

Pharmacy and Chemistry (CPC) to provide "the Association with an agency capable of testing the claims and contents of proprietary medicines" sold to doctors, and later, of patent medicines in general.[83] A laboratory for the purpose was established in late 1906. The council's reports became a regular feature in *JAMA* and were eventually published as a book, *The Propaganda for Reform*, which appeared in several editions. This did not halt the flood of proprietaries, however, and with new ones coming on the market all the time, some of them potentially convenient and perhaps even medically valuable, the AMA reluctantly acknowledged that commercial remedies were a fact of modern medical life and decided to provide the profession with a means to sort those that were acceptable from those that were not. The rules for acceptable products were published in 1905.[84]

To be approved by the CPC, a proprietary item had to name its active ingredients and provide the chemical composition of its formula; it could not be advertised to the public (unless it was a disinfectant, cosmetic, or food); its label and any literature the patient would see could not identify the diseases for which the article might be used; the claims made on its behalf could not be "unwarranted, exaggerated, or misleading." The evaluations began to appear in *JAMA* shortly after the council was formed; in 1907, approved items were publicized in the first edition of *New and Nonofficial Remedies*. In the meantime, Wiley's Pure Food and Drug Act, passed in early 1906 by a Congress for whom the voice of an outraged public was now louder than that of the nostrum lobby, was signed into law by Theodore Roosevelt on 30 June and went into effect 1 January 1907.[85] Administered by the Bureau of Chemistry in the Department of Agriculture, the law created a short list of specific items (including alcohol, morphine, opium, heroin, and acetanilid and its derivatives) that were required to appear on the labels of concoctions that contained them. Failure to list them could result in a charge of misbranding. As a result, some nostrum companies simply went out of business rather than change their recipes or reveal that their "safe and wholesome" products contained cocaine or large quantities of alcohol. Some manufacturers switched from acetanilid to acetphenetidin (Phenacetin) (which was not specified in the label law), but by 1914 the courts declared this was a derivative of acetanilid and therefore needed to be listed. Because acetphenetidin was always costlier than acetanilid, many nostrum companies decided to keep their old recipes and carry on as before. Nevertheless, the Pure Food and Drug Act was greeted as true progress, saving American men, women, and children from an early grave. It also, in a sense, saved the AMA, which in the wake of the act emerged rejuvenated and energetic. The increase in subscriptions to *JAMA* and in membership in the AMA suggests that the organization's message was in fact finding a growing audience among doctors; many historians mark the rise of the AMA as *the* authoritative voice of American medicine from this period.[86]

But if medical authority is in any way measured by the control of drugs, then the AMA (or doctors in general, for that matter) still had a long road to travel. The Pure Food and Drug Act was simply a label law. It did not give any privileges to physicians, did not restrict any drugs for use by prescription only, and did not prevent Americans from continuing to treat themselves with any medicine they chose. The law did not even address the question of extravagant or misleading advertising and could not penalize a nostrum for claiming that it cured cancer, tuberculosis, or bad blood. The Sherley amendment of 1912 attempted to correct this but was in fact ineffective because it was premised on intent: if prosecutors could not prove that the proprietor knew his claims were false, there was no fraud. All the drug's owner had to do was swear he believed in his product. A physician's opinion to the contrary had no standing.[87]

The 1906 law may have caused the nostrum business to pause for a moment, but the trade recovered quickly. The Proprietary Association of America, which at first had been quite alarmed by the muckrakers, now saw that its fears were largely unfounded, and the number of companies in the PAA actually rose from 145 in 1896 to 254 by 1914.[88] Stung by the sharp criticism, however, and sensitive to the public mood, the PAA thought it prudent to begin its own public relations campaign to restore respectability to its products. Paradoxically, the new law helped: nostrums were safer than ever, the association said, now that the labels would indicate the presence of the alcohol, narcotics, or acetanilid that the muckrakers had demonized. Furthermore, alert to the public's increasing concern about narcotics addiction, the PAA wanted it known that their organization was now (and always had been) "in favor of getting legislation to regulate the sale of narcotic drugs," but the industry also wanted to emphasize that its products were now (and always had been) safe.[89] In a booklet (*Facts Worth*

Knowing) that the PAA distributed around the country, statistics were presented that disputed the role of nostrums in causing all the deaths that
had been attributed to them.[90] A few years later the PAA contemplated creating a two-reel motion picture to record the scientific and hygienic production of a proprietary medicine. (The Lydia Pinkham Company was
suggested as the "star," but unfortunately the production does not appear
to have materialized.)[91] An industry that had been worth $74.5 million in
1905 alone could scarcely be expected to give up without a fight.[92] Consequently, nostrums flourished much as before (although with fewer narcotics, perhaps), continued to promise death-defying cures, and continued
to entice millions of Americans to buy them. By the PAA's own estimate,
the business was worth $142 million in 1909. According to Frank Cheney,
president of the PAA, this was clear proof that the public had more confidence in remedies that were attested to by "ten thousand testimonials"
than in those that came from the uncertainties of medical science.[93]

The AMA itself, in fact, did not consider the new law much of a triumph, simply a hopeful step in the right direction.[94] The first federal legislation that actually gave physicians control over an important class of
drugs was passed shortly after, however, reinforcing the regulatory trend
and the growth of medical authority. Established largely in reaction to the
increasing fears of addiction (or, more likely, of addicts) in American society, the Harrison Narcotic Act of 1914 required that most opiates be
restricted to prescriptions written for valid medical reasons, effectively
curtailing self-treatment with large amounts of these drugs. Although this
law gave physicians authority over what had been a traditional right of
self-medication, doctors were not altogether happy with it. It required a
good deal of record keeping, and failure to comply with the new statutes
could turn both physicians and pharmacists into criminals. Exuberant officials who did not think addiction was a valid medical condition sent some
doctors to jail to make their point.[95]

At any rate, neither the Food and Drug Act nor the Harrison Narcotic
Act addressed, far less resolved, the equally important problem of physicians' proprietary prescribing. Reformers still hoped that on-going im-
provements in medical education would eventually bear fruit, but in the
meantime the pages of *JAMA* kept up the antiproprietary campaign, deleting offending advertisements and urging other medical publications to do

the same.[96] *JAMA* received praise from other editors because its policies would force "the concealed journalistic supporters of the nostrum traffic" into the open.[97] "Beyond the inherent difficulties of the task," said the *Boston Medical and Surgical Journal*, "we can conceive of no possible objection to the plan."[98] But those "inherent difficulties" were in fact insurmountable for publications that depended for their survival on the revenue from proprietary advertisers. The *New York Medical Journal*, for example, approved of the AMA's intentions in principle but anticipated difficulties from vendors. *JAMA* at least had other income from membership dues and could afford to be noble.[99] Advertising income remained crucial to most journals, whatever the views of the AMA.[100] Therefore very few joined *JAMA* in actively campaigning against the "nostrum evil." Although they deplored doctors' overuse of proprietaries, they did not necessarily deplore the proprietaries per se. Even some public health officials thought journal advertising fundamentally a positive thing, otherwise the manufacturers would simply create their own journals or advertise to the public. "Is it not far better to have these dealers under the control of the profession, as they now are, than to force them to look to the people for support?"[101]

In 1908 the *New York Medical Journal* noted that trade names were "convenient protection" for manufacturers' products and that many proprietary formulas had been good enough to be admitted to the *USP*—"always without credit to the originator."[102] The *Massachusetts Medical Journal* thought prescribing from the *Pharmacopoeia* and *National Formulary* was "an excellent suggestion," but proprietary concoctions had the important advantages of being familiar and reliable. What were doctors supposed to substitute for them? So this publication carried not only advertisements for such things as Antiphlogistine and Anasarcin but also brief "reports" in the text pages celebrating the virtues of these medications.[103] One such piece about Antikamnia clearly was meant to suggest that this drug did not possess the side effects associated with acetanilid. The writer described how he had used other antipyretic analgesics "with fear and trembling," concerned for the safety of his patients' hearts: "However, since I have used antikamnia tablets I suffer from no fears on [that] score."[104] In 1912, *JAMA* reported that Antikamnia ("one of the most impudent frauds ever foisted on the medical profession") was still advertised "by more than fifty

American medical journals, ranging from the New York *Medical Record* and the *Annals of Surgery* down."[105] In 1910, Antikamnia had even won the right *not* to list acetphenetidin (which it was using as a substitute for acetanilid) on its label, on the grounds that it was not a derivative of acetanilid. (The government appealed, lost, appealed again, and finally won in 1914.)[106] Despite the special attention that both *JAMA* and Samuel Hopkins Adams had given Antikamnia, the product's career was long and lucrative, disappearing only in 1950.

Despite the confidence in regular doctors that muckrakers had shown, there were many corners of the medical world in which the AMA was not welcome. Many members of the public, although they might seek professional advice in areas in which the new medical science had impressed them (surgery or diphtheria treatment, for example), were still just as likely to ignore physicians when it came to other aspects of their health—especially when self-treatment had proved to be efficacious and inexpensive. The treatment of headaches with headache powders is a case in point. In fact, of all the items targeted by medical and lay muckrakers, the headache powders escaped virtually unscathed. Some drug companies responded to the 1906 law either by lying about the contents or by changing the formula, usually from acetanilid to phenacetin, but acetanilid remained an identified ingredient of many other headache preparations for many more years without hurting sales. The horror stories of death by acetanilid and the depravity of addiction to coal tar medications do not seem to have struck a chord with the laity. It may well be that the new labels were misleading the public into believing "that the government guarantees [the drugs'] harmlessness."[107] But Americans had already used these drugs extensively for two decades, and they simply did not consider them to be particularly dangerous—certainly not as dangerous as narcotics or alcohol. So long as these remedies were an effective way to treat headaches, the public was not inclined to give them up.

The AMA responded by reprinting Adams's *Collier's* articles in book form and in general by maintaining a higher public profile with respect to questions of drug use. But if the AMA could not control what ads appeared in medical journals, it had even less chance of controlling what ads the public saw in newspapers and other media, and no chance of controlling the rate of consumption. Acetanilid-based headache powders remained best sellers. In 1907, the *Druggists Circular* reported that enough acetanilid was used every year in the United States to "give every man woman and child in the country an average of ten adult doses."[108] Accounts of "appalling" habitual use of headache remedies "almost as much as morphine and cocaine" appeared in the press long after the act went into effect, with the rise in heart disease again being attributed to the use of these coal tar medications.[109] Stearns Headache Cure, one of the popular culprits, apparently was promoted extensively in the New York City subway system.[110] As we saw earlier, however, headache powders were just as likely to be publicized by druggists as by any other means. According to one survey, "almost every pharmacist [prepared] a remedy to replace the 'patent' articles."[111] Drugstore windows were "fairly yellow with . . . displays" of powders and tablets.[112]

The nation's pharmacists had in fact not shown much enthusiasm for the Pure Food and Drug Act or the AMA's antinostrum campaign. Their overwhelming concerns at the turn of the century were price-cutting (that is, selling name brands at less than the usual rates) and other retail matters, and they gave more of their attention to the National Association of Retail Druggists (NARD, formed in 1898) than to the APhA.[113] An antinostrum stance was simply unrealistic. Prominent members of the APhA of course endorsed the bill's intentions, but many pharmaceutical periodicals barely discussed the matter, not wishing to upset the manufacturers of the patent medicines that were so crucial to most pharmacists' livelihoods.[114] At any rate, with or without a label law, retail pharmacies would still be selling proprietaries. Some pharmacists now even defended patent medicines as a legitimate part of the trade. The *Bulletin of Pharmacy*, for example, called Edward Bok's antinostrum editorials in the *Ladies' Home Journal* "rabid" and thought "many of the charges brought against proprietary articles by the reformers [had] very little basis in reason." Bok's belief that nostrums promoted alcoholism was ridiculous, said the *Bulletin*, given that the medicines were meant to be consumed by the spoonful, not by the glass, although the journal did think the stand against cocaine snuff, "the greatest and perhaps only serious evil" of the patent medicine industry, was a good thing.[115] Journals with strong ties to the PAA, such as the *National Druggist*, were even more supportive of proprietaries and the public's right to choose what it ingested. (At the same time, the editor proclaimed that secret formulas were "property rights . . . recognized and protected by every civilized nation on earth, and by every class of individuals, except anarchists, communists, and this bumptious Council [of the AMA].")[116]

Pharmacists were certainly not indifferent to the problems associated with the headache remedies. As early as the turn of the century, some drug journals were already expressing concern about overuse of the powders and sometimes reminded druggists that "It is not for pharmacists to say what constitutes a safe headache remedy. [We] should leave the practice of medicine to those qualified to engage in it."[117] Other pharmacists were a little less rigorous and argued that over-the-counter headache remedies had their place. There was even a kind of protocol: When a customer demanded a brand-name remedy, the proprietor should sell it. If the request was for "something good," this was an excellent opportunity to sell the house brand. But a desperate appeal for "anything" because nothing so far had worked was a different matter. In this case druggists were advised to send the patient to a physician and "at least try to tell him that something more than a headache [ailed] him."[118]

Headache remedies (still largely consisting of acetanilid, acetphenetidin, or sometimes Antipyrine, labeled or not) remained a very large part of the retail drug business. One pharmacist in 1912 estimated that a colleague dispensed "about a thousand 3 ½-grain acetanilide tablets per month," whereas his own store had sold four thousand ten-cent headache remedy packages, seven hundred boxes of cold cures, and fifteen pounds of bulk remedy (total profits, $400).[119] It is possible, of course, that some of these were dispensed on the orders of physicians, but the fact that this particular author did not think these sales were wise—the coal tar drugs, in his view, although he still sold them, were too hazardous—suggests that the purchasers were mostly self-medicators. But so long as they were making their purchases in a drugstore, there was some prospect that customers could be directed to other products or to their doctors and that the pharmacists could guarantee the contents of whatever they sold. Druggists, after all, were not merely shopkeepers. They, too, were guardians of public welfare and, like physicians, claimed the appropriate professional expertise for the role.[120]

By 1900, headache powders had become well-established articles in great demand by the public, available as national or private brands in any pharmacy. The 1906 law affected this situation very little. Even the publicity given to the hazards of acetanilid does not seem to have quelled the public's appetite, as the sales figures bear out. It was druggists, not doctors, who were the de facto gatekeepers for what were state-of-the-art medications and who—unlike many physicians—were willing to respond immediately to a headache pain by providing an effective painkiller. Rather than submit to the cost and delay of dealing with physicians (who might only prescribe a laxative anyway), the public voted with its feet, as it were, and took its headache business to the drugstore. Headache remedies required professional skill to formulate and were profitable besides; druggists had no intention of giving them up. Neither did the proprietary firms.[121]

Rapid and efficacious headache treatment was now firmly established in the domestic camp and was a profitable sideline for druggists and manufacturers alike, with every indication that despite side effects and other problems, the aniline-based powders would have a long career ahead of them. Yet within a few years, a new drug would eclipse them all—in profits, in quantities consumed, and in being inextricably linked to headaches. The drug, of course, was Aspirin.

6

The Bayer Company

Drugs as Big Business

Aspirin first appeared in the spring of 1899 in a handful of articles in a few German medical journals.[1] The authors introduced it without fanfare as a serviceable substitute for the salicylic acid and sodium salicylate that had been in use for more than twenty years to treat rheumatic disorders. Aspirin reduced fever and inflammation quickly, but more importantly it did not appear to wreak havoc on the stomach. Side effects were minimal. Patients tolerated it quite well. They did not rebel against the treatment. The doctors who tested it and the company that manufactured it therefore recommended the drug as a promising antirheumatic medication and no doubt expected respectable profits from its use in this modest market. No one, however, apparently anticipated that in less than two decades this new compound would become the manufacturer's best-selling medicine and the world's most widely used drug (a distinction it still holds), not so much because of its role in treating rheumatism but because of its effectiveness in managing minor pain, especially headaches. And by the time Aspirin's overall popularity was apparent, it was also apparent that it had achieved this exalted status not simply because of its considerable medical merits but also because of the deliberate business policies and practices of its manufacturer, the Farbenfabriken vormals Friedrich Bayer und Companie of Elberfeld, Germany.

From the first, Bayer's activities as provider of valuable medications had irritated members of the medical professions in the United States because it seemed to embody all the sins they had already seen in American firms. Bayer in fact became a prominent example of what critics of a commercialized drug industry had feared. Profits came first. Physicians were a market to be manipulated. Pharmacists were merely sales agents. Truth in advertising was optional. Manufacturers had far more control over drugs than doctors did. Observing these flaws in American companies, reformers had long been advocating pharmacopeial prescribing and boycotts as the best solutions. But Bayer was not really comparable to most American drug makers. Its products were not available from any other company (at least, not legally). Doctors who wished to use the most up-to-date, science-based medications, endorsed by the world's most eminent medical men, had no choice but to patronize Bayer—a foreign company, moreover. To many people in the United States, this situation was infuriating and intolerable. The passions it aroused came to a head with Aspirin. But Aspirin was not the first popular Bayer headache remedy to provoke the ire of the American medical world: Phenacetin had already tested the waters. How Bayer handled these two important drugs and how doctors, pharmacists, and the public reacted had profound implications for the drug industry as a whole, for the image and authority of the professions— and especially for headache victims who had discovered that these two Bayer medications provided particularly good relief.

Bayer was not a traditional drug maker with roots in either pharmacy or medicine and had not been founded by idealists who longed to alleviate human suffering. Rather, it was a very successful synthetic dyestuffs manufacturer that had already become one of the largest chemical producers in the world by the time it began making drugs in the mid-1880s. Competitive, aggressive, and fiercely protective of its property rights, Bayer was under no illusion that its forays into medicines would be any less commercial than its experiences with its dyes. With its reputation for scientific achievement and high-quality products, however, the company had no difficulty in defining itself as ethical, and therefore it did not advertise to the public. Good rapport with physicians was always one of its principal concerns. Yet it ignored virtually all the other criteria for ethical drugs, especially those related to trade names and patents: "from the beginning, the sale of its pharmaceutical products became a business in proprietary articles."[2]

In the beginning, though, Bayer did not quite understand how to exploit the drug market, and with its first drug, acetphenetidin, the company did not act quickly enough to maintain complete control of its product. Unable to obtain a German patent on the chemical, Bayer nevertheless coined the trade name Phenacetin and advertised Phenacetin-Bayer. Almost immediately, other German firms began manufacturing their own phenacetin (Phenacetin-Riedel, Phenacetin-Hoechst), using Bayer's trade name as a generic term. When the drug entered the German pharmacopoeia in 1890 as phenacetin, it was too late for Bayer to reclaim the word. In Germany, at least, the term had become public property, and as a result, Bayer's European profits from this drug were less than it had hoped.[3] Nevertheless, medical chemicals seemed to be a promising sideline, so in 1896 the company established a pharmaceutical research laboratory that, over the next decade or so, produced a small pool of useful medicinal products, some of which became quite popular—heroin, for example. Most did not become very profitable, however, because they did not meet the stringent criteria for a German patent and so were in constant competition with other companies' versions. Consequently, Bayer and the other drug manufacturers often agreed to share the market so that all might have a piece of the pie, but this was not a satisfactory solution. Pricing agreements still kept profit margins low. There was one market, however, in which Bayer did not have to share its products with anyone at all, and where the profits were accordingly much higher—the United States.[4]

The U.S. patent laws for chemicals were different from the laws of most other countries. A U.S. patent was often granted to the product, not the process that created it, which meant that whoever arrived first at the patent office with evidence of a new chemical could get a monopoly on that substance for seventeen years, regardless of how many other cheaper or better methods of production might be invented subsequently. The chemical itself only went into the public domain when the patent expired. Bayer was thus able to obtain patents for virtually all the drugs it sold in the United States, even those it had to share in Germany.[5] In making the most of this situation, the company became a conspicuous example of what advantages (and, rather unexpectedly, what disadvantages) could result from such secure monopolies.

As a newcomer to the American ethical market in the late 1880s, Bayer chose to be represented by a veteran sales agency, W. H. Schieffelin and

Company of New York, one of the oldest drug manufacturing and whole-saling establishments in the country. Apparently Bayer selected the company for its experience and integrity.[6] Although a member of the Proprietary Association, Schieffelin also had its own ethical product lines and accordingly advertised Bayer's drugs only to the pharmaceutical and medical professions. The ads were conspicuous and numerous, appearing in large numbers of professional periodicals on a regular basis. Initially they were rather text-heavy and not particularly attractive, but they quickly became eye-catching and appealing. The products themselves (Phenacetin and the sedative Sulfonal were the first two to be marketed) became very popular, perhaps because of the advertising but also because of their clinical success. Phenacetin in fact became an immediate and sus-tained best seller, accounting for 50 percent of Bayer's drug sales in America before 1906. Even better, as early as 1895 Phenacetin was one of the most frequently prescribed drugs in the country.[7] Schieffelin appeared to be doing a wonderful job on behalf of the German firm.

Yet all was not well between Bayer and its sales agent. Drug sales had in fact declined by the mid-1890s, prompting Bayer in 1896 to ask Dr. Hugo Schweitzer, a German-American chemist living in New York, to investi-gate.[8] Bayer also hired Schweitzer to be head of the American pharmaceu-tical division, and his fact-finding tour of the country turned up some rather disturbing information: American druggists disliked Schieffelin intensely. Bayer products were expensive, and pharmacists believed (erro-neously) that this was because Schieffelin owned Bayer's patent, which allowed the jobber to buy "Phenacetine from Bayer at German market prices and then [extort] a high price in America."[9] Schweitzer learned that druggists were even willing to boycott Schieffelin so that it "would soon have to give up the agency," which would then prevent it from making "so enormous a profit with Bayer's articles." There was some justification for the pharmacists' anger: an ounce of acetphenetidin that cost six cents in Germany and fifteen cents in Canada cost one dollar in the United States. Because markups were lower with branded products, pharmacists' in-comes were adversely affected. The solution that a number of druggists resorted to, however, was illegal: smuggling the drug from Canada.

It was not Schieffelin, of course, that had set the prices but Bayer. Schieffelin had even asked Bayer to price Phenacetin at no more than thirty

cents per ounce—twice what Bayer got in Canada and a little more than
Antifebrin sold for—to mollify the nation's druggists, but "the Bayer directors refused, and in 1896 . . . voted 'to defend our good rights until the last,
and receive the full benefit from our valuable patents.'"[10] At any rate, as of
June 1898, Schieffelin was no longer the agent for the Farbenfabriken of
Elberfeld Company in the United States.[11] Bayer now began to market its
drugs itself, at which point Americans discovered that the prices would
remain high, even after Bayer began to manufacture drugs at its plant in
Rensselaer, New York, in about 1903.[12] For many pharmacists, smuggling and
the use of contraband now became something of a patriotic duty as they
sought to undermine Bayer's monopolies. Popular as both a prescription
and domestic drug, Phenacetin was the principal commodity in question.

Some druggists, in all innocence, apparently bought cheaper Bayer
Phenacetin in Canada or Europe and brought it home to sell, not intending
to break any laws. They were dumbfounded when customs officers told
them that it was illegal for them even to swallow the drug, far less resell it,
in the United States. Government agents seized the goods on behalf of the
patent holder, at which point, presumably, they should have been returned to Bayer or destroyed. But officials seemed unclear on this point,
and in several instances the confiscated goods were put up for auction.
Dealers bought them at bargain rates (10 percent of the value), obviously
expecting to re-sell them somewhere in the world for a healthy profit—
until they discovered that Bayer would bring an action against them if they
tried.[13] One Rhode Island company found itself the unhappy owner of five
thousand ounces of Phenacetin with which it could do absolutely nothing.[14] Although it was the genuine Bayer product, made by the Bayer firm,
it had come into the United States illegally and any further use of it violated Bayer's property rights. Other "imports" of Phenacetin, of course,
were not so innocent and were deliberate attempts to get around Bayer's
monopoly and high prices. But as far as Bayer was concerned, the smuggling problem was to be resolved not by conciliatory pricing but by litigation. In this the company was adamant.

Battle lines were thus drawn between Farbenfabriken Bayer and a significant segment of America's pharmacists who were willing to break the
law to show their deep displeasure with the company. (And it was not just
high prices that made them unhappy. Bayer also was contributing to the

prepackaged pills, tablets, and capsules—*Originalartikeln*—that were de-skilling the pharmaceutical profession.) At times the situation took on the atmosphere of a comic opera: once, a German sailor who secreted goods on his person aroused the suspicion of inspectors, who "had been struck by [his] abnormal size."[15] In another case, "packages were found under the stiff derby hat" worn by a smuggler apprehended by the Detroit police.[16] The goods being smuggled were supplied by Canadian dealers, who were providing American jobbers with genuine Phenacetin from which they had removed Bayer's labels that stated the product could not be re-sold in the United States.[17] One Mr. A. C. Smith became infamous for engaging in this trafficking, assisted in the enterprise by his wife, who was arrested when agents found two hundred dollars worth of Phenacetin in her rooms in Detroit. Mr. Smith, having had a previous run-in with the law for dealing in illegal Phenacetin, "absconded to Canada," leaving his wife, Elsie, "a handsome little brunette probably not more than 19 years old . . . weeping in [the marshal's] office all . . . afternoon."[18] We are not told whether she ever rejoined her husband, but a few months later Mr. Smith was sending out postcards from Windsor, Ontario, advising American druggists that he was prepared to supply them with Bayer drugs at prices well below what they cost in the United States. He was still in business in Windsor five years later, ranting about "certain New York parties [that] have endeavored to monopolize the trade in these various products and, by use of the courts, of unfair laws and of a private detective force, to stamp out all competition and are asking an outrageous price for these chemicals, considering their REAL value." Good druggists opposed such monopolies, he said. One can imagine him shaking his fist in righteous indignation as he looked across the Detroit River at those unfortunate Americans forced to suffer such outrages.[19]

Bayer was unmoved by these sentiments and vigorously pursued cases of Phenacetin smuggling and infringement whenever and wherever they occurred. In one instance the company spent six months ferreting out information about a gang operating in Cincinnati.[20] One smuggler in Detroit even worked in the packing department of Parke-Davis. (Given that Hugo Schweitzer had once accused Parke-Davis itself of smuggling Phenacetin, this may be significant.)[21] Most infractions seem to have been punished by injunctions or fines, but some offenders went to jail. One elderly man—a German chemist who said he was down on his luck—was

sentenced to sixty days plus a fine of a thousand dollars.[22] Another man
was sentenced to a year in the penitentiary.[23] Because the ultimate leaders
of these smuggling operations were fewer in number and more difficult to
identify and apprehend than the druggists who ended up with the contraband, Bayer devoted a good deal of energy to punishing the pharmacists,
getting the names of the culprits from the smugglers in return for amnesty.
Between 1895 and 1906, Bayer threatened some seven thousand druggists
with prosecution for violating its property rights and actually filed suit
against eight hundred or so.[24]

The pharmaceutical press was up in arms over these activities, but the
law was on Bayer's side.[25] Bayer owned the Phenacetin patent and had
every right to prosecute individuals who trespassed, although as the historian Thomas Reimer has pointed out, public opinion in the Progressive era
did not favor monopolies, and it was not impossible that the courts might
eventually side with the pharmacists. Bayer had the resources and the
willpower to sustain lengthy litigation, however, and most attempts to
challenge its position went nowhere. The Chicago Retail Druggists Association, for example, which had based its challenge of Bayer on the antitrust
laws, gave up in 1897 and agreed to recognize the Phenacetin patent, even
though a judge in the case was not unsympathetic to the pharmacists'
point of view.[26] Another case, which began in 1898 when a dealer tried to
challenge the validity of the patent itself, was not resolved until May 1901,
when the judge—in this case showing no sympathy for the pharmacists'
cause—decided in favor of Bayer, even calling the company "the benefac-
tors of mankind."[27] "This decision in substance is a very complete victory
for the phenacetine people," bemoaned the *Pharmaceutical Era*, which had
been trying from the start to rally support and raise money for the dealer's
legal fees.[28] But the *Era* was pleased to note several months later that an
infringement case in Chicago had ended quickly with Bayer paying the
costs, even though the drugstore in question was enjoined from selling
phenacetin. Bayer got what it wanted, but the "settlement . . . [bore] the
aspects of a victory for the Chicago firm, who [was] to be congratulated
upon having at least fought a drawn battle."[29] Legally, however, Bayer was
still holding all the cards. American courts had declared its property rights
sacrosanct, and druggists who violated them were criminals. Still, many
druggists remained defiant. Smuggling, in fact, "became much worse,"

with a significant number of pharmacists now abandoning their cloak-and-dagger amateurism and instead patronizing "professionals such as Louis Fulmer, a renegade druggist, whose gang of several dozen men and women carried Bayer drugs from Windsor, Ontario, to Detroit, from which they were mailed all over the country."[30]

For the most part, American druggists justified these illegal activities as a fight against immoral foreign monopolies and unconscionably high prices. They had also obtained the tacit approval of the medical profession and the public, who at least did not comment much on the situation, one way or another. Doctors, at any rate, had their own objections to Bayer's behavior and were not inclined to be sympathetic to the company. But the nature of smuggling also attracted a disreputable element. More and more frequently, illicit Phenacetin turned out to be acetanilid or worse—talcum powder. Such revelations cast Bayer not as villain but as victim, whose reputation for quality products was being harmed by unscrupulous ruffians. Harmed, too, was the public, poisoned by who-knew-what in counterfeits from who-knew-where. Bayer publicists sent accounts of these frauds to newspapers around the country. To pharmacy publications it sent reminders that Bayer would "PROSECUTE ALL INFRINGERS OF OUR RIGHTS" as well as requests that editors remind their readers of the penalties for smuggling and counterfeiting, and the hazards of buying from spurious dealers. Bayer asked that feature articles on these topics coincide with special Bayer advertisements.[31] (No publication with an anti-Bayer editorial record, by the way, seems to have ever refused to take Bayer advertising.) As the instances of counterfeiting increased, journals such as the *Pharmaceutical Era* reluctantly advised readers to buy only from reputable persons but nonetheless regretted the circumstances that had compelled so many American druggists to break the law. They also regretted that the publicity generated by counterfeiting cases was often sensationalized in the daily press, as when the headline "Poisoned by a Bogus Drug" appeared over an article in the *Boston Traveler*, which described the near-death experience of a man who had consumed adulterated phenacetin.[32] Newspapers in fact were making more frequent references to "dangerous gangs of counterfeiters," even implying that many pharmacists deliberately bought cheaper, substandard materials in order to increase their profit margins. To pharmacists, this was yet another insult to a beleaguered profession.

Gradually, however, as solid evidence of widespread pharmaceutical wrongdoing accumulated, eventually coinciding with the muckraking campaigns on behalf of the food and drug bill, Bayer's efforts began to bear fruit. In 1902, the New York City's Board of Health bought 373 samples of Phenacetin from city druggists suspected of dealing with illicit suppliers and found that 315 of them were adulterated or contaminated.[33] When a Bayer investigation in 1904 convincingly demonstrated that some five thousand druggists in New York state had bought fraudulent Bayer drugs from one particular shady operator, the New York State Medical Society— now publicly horrified at the druggists' behavior—abandoned its moral support of the pharmacists and offered to help Bayer instead. Then in 1905 the influential but Chicago-based National Association of Retail Druggists (NARD) finally conceded that these extralegal practices were not just a New York problem but were detrimental to both the public welfare and the reputation of professional pharmacists throughout the country. It began a campaign of its own against Mr. A. C. Smith, who was still residing in Windsor, Ontario, but who was now quite notorious and quite incensed by NARD's claim that his Phenacetin was adulterated.[34]

Such publicity was not good for the smuggling business, however. Nor was humiliation or possible criminal charges worth the risk to professional pharmacists if they were caught with counterfeits, now that the public had become concerned with these matters. Druggists should only deal in brand names from reputable dealers. Bayer's persistence had paid off. Not only had it convincingly argued for its property rights (for which there was in fact very little sympathy), but it had also taken the moral high road. It was not an avaricious foreign manufacturer that had put Americans at risk with substandard or poisonous products but ignorant, lazy, or greedy American pharmacists. In this instance, at least, the company's mercantile interest in its monopoly rights was not at odds with public safety. To the dismay of many of its critics, Bayer had demonstrated the advantages of industrial drugs: factory-packaged, premeasured, and scientifically super- vised, they were safer, more accurate, and less prone to unauthorized sub- stitution than were the old-fashioned, haphazard, and potentially harmful concoctions dispensed by the average, perhaps inadequately trained (and maybe even dishonest) druggist. Furthermore, Bayer had kept its prices high not simply as a matter of greed but as an indication of quality—a fea-

ture of Bayer's genuine products that no one had ever faulted. Only when
the patent expired in 1906 did Bayer, in a "spirit of comity," finally reduce
the price of its Phenacetin to a more competitive (but still high) thirty-
three cents per ounce, gambling that dealers would rather pay more for
Bayer's reputation than risk buying cheaper versions (at about a dollar per
pound) from such chemical manufacturers as the St. Louis firms of Monsanto and Mallinckrodt, which had no previous experience with this
chemical.[35] These American companies themselves gambled that the market for the drug would remain profitably large. All manufacturers were in
fact optimistic that because the Pure Food and Drug Act had not named
acetphenetidin in its list of drugs requiring labels, the headache powder
industry therefore would flock to acetphenetidin producers for an ingredient to replace acetanilid. But only Bayer would be able to sell the drug
under the name Phenacetin—at least, that is what Bayer hoped. The company had no intention of giving up the trade name just because the patent
had expired. Trademark law allowed perpetual ownership. The medical
communities, on the other hand, were anxious to see the word enter the
public domain. Bayer's efforts to retain this particular property thus
served to keep the relationship between the company and the druggists on
the boil.

From the start, Bayer (and the other German firms) had advertised,
reported on, and published about their medicinal products only in terms
of their trade names, to the great annoyance of the medical elites but without objection from the rank and file, who "generally consider[ed] such
brand names as synonyms of the pharmacopoeial articles and use[d] them
in this sense."[36] The records of a Wisconsin druggist for 1893 and 1894, for
example, reveal many orders for phenacetin, antifebrin, and antikamnia
(uncapitalized), a few for acetanilid, but none for acetphenetidin, and certainly none for phenyldimethylpyrazolone. Ten years later, a Milwaukee
druggist filled similar prescriptions and had at least one order for
phenacetinum, the Latinized form suggesting very strongly that the prescriber considered the word to be a generic term.[37] Bayer reinforced this
perception (perhaps inadvertently at first, simply copying its European
practice) with advertisements that almost always proclaimed its product
as Phenacetin-Bayer, which could suggest that only the company name
Bayer was proprietary. As a result, American doctors wrote "phenacetin" in

their prescriptions just as they would use "cod liver oil," unaware that they were prescribing by trade name. Pharmacists were more likely to know the difference between the brand and the generic designation but were obligated by the patent and by the prohibition on substitution to dispense the Bayer drug anyway. As one New York druggist noted, "The manufacturers . . . have tried, and in many instances successfully tried, to confound the minds of the medical profession, the press and the public" on the question of generic and brand-name identity.[38]

The status of the German trade names was a very current topic around the beginning of the century. In fact, the eighth decennial revision of the *United States Pharmacopoeia* in 1900 (*USP* VIII) was going to address this very issue, because one of its tasks was to provide the official or generic names of drugs in general use.[39] As one of the most popular items under discussion (and with its patent about to expire in 1906), Phenacetin would be a test case. Through the sixth revision (1880), all items under consideration had had public names as a matter of course, because all drugs were assumed to be in the public domain and none was exclusively artificial. Until the seventh revision in 1890, revision committees had maintained a strictly ethical position that simply refused to admit any drug with a patent or a trade name, no matter how popular it might be. Thus, in 1890 acetanilid was admitted but Phenacetin and Antipyrine (and the name Antifebrin) were not. Ten years later, however, the pharmacopeial committee could no longer ignore the fact that more and more proprietary or synthetic drugs had a place in professional medical practice. It was generally—although not universally—conceded that the *USP* should in some way recognize these chemical entities, despite their patents. The AMA, for example, finally resolved at its annual meeting in 1899 that its delegates to the revision committee of 1900 would advocate inclusion of synthetics "of definite and known chemical structure without regard to patents."[40] But what names they should have remained a sticking point.

The chair of the revision committee, Charles Rice, stated his view from the outset, asserting that "the only practical solution of this difficulty" was to provide the chemicals with both their scientific and their commercial names.[41] When committee discussions got under way in 1900, carried on by long-distance correspondence, this position seemed to be the one most members favored. One correspondent, for example, noted that because prescribers would never learn to use the scientific names of these drugs ("which, by the way, in some cases would take up more than one line of text"), it was mere common sense to include the trade names in the publication.[42] Another correspondent hoped that the inclusion of trade names would "legally make every such name public property. The Proprietors will no longer have any right to claim the names as Trade-Marks." Another member, on the other hand, was reluctant to approve the inclusion of drugs that were part of the "systematic robbery of the medical profession of our country . . . carried on by the manufacturers of synthetic remedies."[43] There were fears that the owners would not, in fact, lose their rights to the trade names, and *USP* recognition of their property would give them an unfair advantage. Even though the drugs in question were few in number, they were "likely to give us much embarrassment in the future," according to Joseph Remington, who became chairman after Rice's untimely death in 1901, and was less accommodating on this question than his predecessor had been.[44] By early 1904, opinion was divided between using a Latinized form of the trade name (thus, phenacetinum) or inventing a short, scientific name, as the British had done for phenyldimethylpyrazolone, calling it phenazonum rather than antipyrinum. Nevertheless, one correspondent noted that he did "not see how we can avoid adopting the trade-name in some instances. . . . [It] should be employed as a synonym, or mentioned somewhere in the text." Because the coined scientific name was new and unfamiliar, said another member, readers would not "know where to find what they [were] looking for" if there were no cross-reference with the trade name.[45] Despite these points, in July 1904 the committee rejected all forms of trade names and adopted strictly scientific terminology (although Antipyrine slipped in as antipyrina). Henceforth, phenacetin was to be known as acetphenetidin, despite at least one objection that the word was not easy to spell or pronounce.[46]

The term acetphenetidin had at any rate appeared in the literature from time to time and was not entirely unknown to the medical communities. But *USP* VIII also included three other popular German products, none of which appeared under familiar titles, even as cross-references in the index. For two of these drugs the committee itself had invented names that it said reflected the chemical nature of the compounds, although neither of them bore any resemblance to the trade names under which they

had been advertised and prescribed for nearly twenty years. Readers looking for the sedative Trional could never hope to find it in the *USP* unless
they knew that its new short name was sulphonethylmethane or that it was
cross-referenced in the index as diethylsulphonemethylethylmethane—
not to be confused, by the way, with sulphonmethane or dimethylsul-
phonedimethylmethane, better known as Sulfonal, the other popular
sedative.[47] (The third drug was Aristol, which was entered as thymol iodide.)

Not all members of the committee were happy with the *USP*'s solutions: there was one complaint that these new drug names were not attractive and that "patent articles [would] be ordered as now." Others argued
that the new terms were unscientific and not helpful to either prescribers
or dispensers.[48] But reviews in the medical and pharmaceutical press generally had high praise for the publication overall, even if there were some
reservations about the usefulness of the *USP* in such rapidly changing
times, when manufacturers were supplying novelties to the profession
long before a revision committee got round to evaluating them.[49] In fact,
the *Medical News* declared that the new revision—already obsolete—pan-
dered to commercial interests and was "unworthy of posing as an official
standard."[50] The *Druggists Circular* pointed out something else: the most
questionable aspects of *USP* nomenclature (for Trional, Sulfonal, Phenacetin, and Aristol) involved the products of only one manufacturer—Bayer.
The *Circular* hinted broadly at a conspiracy. By providing the medical community with official generic names, the *USP* had in fact preserved and reinforced the owners' exclusive rights to the trade names. If doctors could
now choose between the terms *phenacetin* and *acetphenetidin*, then their
writing of "phenacetin" in prescriptions would be interpreted to mean it
was definitely the Bayer product they wanted, not acetphenetidin from
Hoechst or Monsanto. Non-Bayer acetphenetidin would still be an illegal
substitution. Pharmacists could still be slapped with lawsuits. "Surely,"
asked the *Circular*, "pharmacists must have begun to wonder how such
strange luck—and always for them good luck—follows this firm. Did they
have a friend upon the committee of revision?"[51] As a result of the *USP*, it
seemed that even without the patent, Bayer was still in firm control of this
product.

No one realistically expected that the run-of-the mill physician, accustomed for twenty years to prescribing the synthetics by trade name, would

substitute *USP* official names, "which the average prescriber will not worry his faculties to remember, much less to write."[52] Besides, doctors had never made much use of the *USP*, considering it more a technical manual for dispensers than a guide for prescribers. The AMA and APhA recommended that doctors at least attempt to discard brand-name use, but physicians could and did claim that they used trade names deliberately, preferring one particular brand over others for good reason.[53] (Regrettably, one of those "good reasons" was that because recent counterfeit scandals had sullied pharmacists' reputations, trademarked, factory-sealed products were more attractive to prescribers.) Nevertheless, most American druggists were hopeful that the courts would see through Bayer's trade-name obfuscations and proclaim the word *phenacetin* generic. But Bayer continued to act as though it had perpetual ownership, claiming that *USP* VIII had settled the name question once and for all.

Privately, however, Bayer was not so confident that it could actually keep the name. Legal precedents were not encouraging (linoleum, for example, had once been a trade name), and the fact that "the name Phenacetin had already been given to the product in the patent" was a troublesome legal blunder that Bayer officials knew would work against the company's interests. At any rate, Bayer seems to have been resigned to the fact that whether or not it kept the name Phenacetin, its share of the market would now be smaller. But it would still be a respectable share because of the large orders from nostrum makers, who would now use acetphenetidin instead of the acetanilid tarnished by the 1906 drug law. "Alas, however, we miscalculated."[54] In 1908, Harvey Wiley interpreted the label law to include acetphenetidin as a derivative of acetanilid, to be treated "in the same manner." It had to be listed on the label, thereby implying that it possessed the same dangers as acetanilid. Despite protests from Bayer, Monsanto, and the Antikamnia Company that acetphenetidin and acetanilid were in no way the same, this interpretation of the law remained in effect. Only one manufacturer chose to replace acetanilid with the far more expensive Bayer product.[55] The other nostrum companies saw no reason to follow suit even with the cheap generic acetphenetidin (which was still more expensive than acetanilid); acetanilid therefore continued to be the chief constituent of headache powders, which, as we have already seen, remained as popular as ever despite the alleged hazards.

As for acetphenetidin, it continued to be an important prescription med-ication, was popular for self-treatment (as it had been before, as Phenacetin), and appeared from time to time in the formulas of various headache remedies.[56] The trade-name situation, however, was never set-tled definitively, although Bayer pursued no more infringement cases after 1906.[57] The company's reputation as a litigant seems to have deterred other firms from using Bayer's term, just to be safe, even though as far as the AMA was concerned, phenacetin (as well as sulfonal and trional) were now all in the public domain.[58] But Bayer was in fact no longer very inter-ested in its once-lucrative drug. The company had another, even more promising new product to which it could turn its attention and to which it gave a patent, a trade name, and the benefit of at least some of the lessons learned from Phenacetin. Aspirin arrived in the United States groomed for success.

The origins and development of Aspirin (acetylsalicylic acid, or ASA) have become the stuff of legend, and although it is an intriguing story and not nearly so straightforward as usually presented, it unfortunately cannot concern us here.[59] It is important to note, however, that Bayer's trade name for its new product was an exceptionally good one. Derived from *acetyl* and *spiraeic* (i.e., salicylic) acid, the term actually represented the components of the compound and was therefore not meaningless—a concession to physicians' concerns. Because it was easy to pronounce in practically all languages, it was therefore easy to remember and to use—a boon for the manufacturers. To some extent the name could make up for Bayer's failure to obtain a German patent, which was really the only negative feature from the company's perspective. Nevertheless, ASA did receive a U.S. patent on 27 February 1900. (It also received a short-lived British patent.) The patent document had been filed several months before the trade name had been invented, so it did not repeat the error Bayer had made with Phenacetin: Letters Patent No. 644,077 was for "acetyl salicylic acid," not Aspirin.

Also, Bayer introduced Aspirin as a therapy for rheumatic disorders, not as a replacement for Phenacetin, which had different and wider appli-cations. Consequently, the initial response to the new drug was limited and sedate but encouraging. In 1902 the *American Journal of Pharmacy* noted that Aspirin was "finding considerable favor" in rheumatic ail-ments.[60] Others praised Aspirin for its antipyretic effects in typhoid fever and tuberculosis, its potential use in diabetes (it seemed to reduce sugar in urine), and its painkilling properties in obstetric cases and even cancer, but because it was a salicylate, its primary applications were in rheumatic conditions, including rheumatic headaches.[61] Yet Aspirin's evident use as a general painkiller contributed to its increasing popularity, to the point that some Americans were tempted once again to challenge Bayer's monopoly. And at only forty-three cents an ounce it was cheaper than Bayer Aspirin in Canada (sixty-five cents). This moderate price was apparently a concession from Bayer to placate pharmacists and forestall smuggling. Nonetheless, generic ASA from Canada at eighteen cents seemed worth the risk to some druggists, who quickly found that Bayer would not tolerate these infractions any more than it had in the case of Phenacetin.

In early 1905, apparently as a test case, Bayer sued a Chicago pharmacist for selling, as Aspirin, ASA he had not purchased from Bayer.[62] Although the Phenacetin precedent had suggested that Bayer would be equally successful with Aspirin suits, the outcome of an Aspirin infringement case in England in July 1905 was a great shock. The Bayer Company in England had sued the Heyden Company for importing ASA into Britain in violation of its patent, but in its defense, Heyden convinced the court that not only had ASA been around long before Bayer had stumbled upon it but that Bayer had been fully aware of this and had been deceptive in its patent specifications. After examining the evidence, the judge agreed, calling the patent "so framed as to obscure the subject as much as possible." He therefore voided the patent—but Bayer was at least allowed to keep the trade name.[63] In the United States, on the other hand, given the outrage that Phenacetin had caused, the loss of the patent might also result in the loss of the trade name—a true calamity. This possibility caused Bayer to approach the American infringement case with considerable trepidation, taking great care to provide convincing evidence that the patent was valid.[64] As it turned out, however, its fears were groundless. In 1909 the judge declared the ASA patent valid for its full legal life, and Bayer was not challenged again on this issue.[65] It kept its monopoly.

Sales of Aspirin increased so dramatically after the decision that the New York office apparently felt it did not have to make a serious effort to advertise. The American office credited Aspirin's success to the path cleared by Phenacetin and Bayer's other popular drugs, and especially to the value of the Bayer name as a guarantee of quality. Consequently the company spent $20,000 less on promotion for all its drugs in 1910 than it had in 1909, and made $185,000 more in sales. It proudly reported this to the German headquarters in the summer of 1911.[66]

Carl Duisberg (Bayer's general manager) and Rudolph Mann (director of the pharmaceutical department in Germany) were astonished at the American office's complacency. "Why," they asked, "did Aspirin for years show only minor progress, and why did . . . the Bayer name not work for other new products? Upon quiet reflection you will find that the huge increase in Aspirin sales can easily find another explanation." It was, they said, the outcome of the patent litigation that forced druggists to buy the brand-name product because they feared prosecution if they did not. Potential infringers might indeed think twice and buy only Bayer, but the ASA patent would not last forever. Competitors would appear. The head office advised New York to pay more attention to the matter.[67] This was timely advice, because the revision committee for *USP* IX had already begun its deliberations for the upcoming publication and Aspirin was on the agenda.

Although whether to admit patented drugs to the pharmacopeia under any name whatsoever was still a topic of much debate, by the time the revision and executive committees began to discuss the issues in detail in 1911, the vast majority of their members were in favor of including acetylsalicylic acid. The comments on Aspirin were neither as numerous nor as passionate as those that had been made about Phenacetin. The decision to admit ASA seemed to be a principled solution that acknowledged the need to set standards for an important medicine but that did not pander to Bayer by acknowledging the trade name.[68] A year later, however, the executive committee voted nine to five against inclusion under any name. The lofty policy that barred commercial substances had apparently won the day, although at least one member had voted "unwillingly" to ban the drug.[69]

This turnabout certainly baffled many onlookers. "Why in the world was [ASA] refused recognition?" asked George Simmons, editor of *JAMA*, writing to the chairman of the executive committee, Joseph Remington. "In any event, the patent expires in 1917. As the next Pharmacopeia will probably remain in force until 1925, there will be eight years in which this product will be common property and yet not mentioned in the Pharmacopeia. It seems to me, therefore that if it is kept out simply because it is patented, it is a very foolish proposition."[70] Remington, however, pointed out that based on the *USP*'s own rules (which no one had yet voted to change), Aspirin could not be admitted. Besides, the policy to refuse recognition to any and all commercial entities was based on admirable principles:

> Would it not be a surrender of these principles to admit Aspirin? . . . being controlled by one house what authority would the Pharmacopoeia have in enforcing its tests for purity? Suppose the Farbenfabriken . . . chose to change or alter the quality of Aspirin in any way, do you suppose they would heed any protest? The Pharmacopoeia would then be in a position of describing one product, the manufacturer would be making another and demanding, under their legal rights, that only the Farbenfabriken Aspirin could be legally used.[71]

Remington had no doubt that Aspirin would continue to be used whether it was in the Pharmacopoeia or not; at least by excluding it, there would be no appearance that the drug or others like it had any sort of official approval.

Not satisfied with this, a number of practitioners continued to argue for inclusion; in mid-1914 the question once again came before the committee.[72] By this time the pendulum had apparently swung back, and the vote was twelve to two to accept Aspirin. But an incident in The Netherlands caused the committee to once again change its mind. The Dutch, who had similar concerns about admitting commercial substances to their own pharmacopeia, had nonetheless entered the term *aspirin* in the belief that the word was legally public. A Dutch drug wholesaler then sold aspirin that had not come from Bayer. Bayer sued. The Dutch courts, perhaps reluctantly, agreed that the law favored the German company and found for the plaintiff. The term Aspirin was Bayer's property alone—pharmacopeia notwithstanding.[73]

The Dutch case highlighted what critics of patented and trademarked drugs had warned would happen in the United States: as long as Bayer remained the word's legal owner, to admit Aspirin to the *USP* would cause great confusion, would expose American druggists to lawsuits, and would

still leave Bayer in complete control of this medicine—"unless we can persuade the owners to give their full consent" to the pharmacopeial use of
the name.[74] It seemed highly unlikely that Farbenfabriken Bayer would
agree to do that. So when *USP* IX was finally published in 1916, there was no
entry for ASA (although it is in the index and on page 504, in a list of
molecular weights and formulas). Acetylsalicylic acid was not officially
admitted until *USP* X was published, in 1924.

Indeed, ever since about 1906, when the Phenacetin patent expired,
Bayer been actively engaged in doing for Aspirin what it had previously
done for Phenacetin: threatening litigation over unauthorized use of the
trade name, identifying and pursuing smugglers, and proclaiming that
millions of Americans were in danger every day because unscrupulous
pharmacists sold them counterfeited and adulterated Aspirin. (Bayer had
help in this campaign from Hoechst, whose syphilis treatment Salvarsan
was also being smuggled or faked.)[75]

Once again, American druggists were offended by the allegations and
saw the whole business as a kind of publicity stunt. The *Pharmaceutical Era*
said that Bayer and Hoechst employed detectives "to seek out sales of substitutes for aspirin" and other patented drugs in an attack that "cannot but
aid the original manufacturers of these preparations in keeping their market."[76] The *Druggists Circular* declared that the companies were prepared to
spend $100,000 on a "crusade" that had as its goal "the wholesale arrest
and punishment of druggists all over the country." The Hoechst representative even alleged that 25 percent of American druggists were guilty of
illegal substitution.[77] Only about half of the four million ounces of Aspirin
sold in the United States annually were the genuine Bayer product, complained the firm's lawyer.[78] The company was convinced that in some parts
of the country (Houston, Texas, for example) up to 75 percent of Aspirin
prescriptions were filled with non-Bayer products.[79] Some of these products came from Canada: Mr. Smith in Windsor was now apparently
"exporting" Aspirin.

Yet with the Phenacetin scandals hardly over, men who were thought
to endanger the health of Americans for the sake of a few cents' profit
could not expect much sympathy. And who knew that they might not also
be engaged in other nefarious activities: in one case, as one pamphlet
exclaimed rather breathlessly, an alleged bootlegger about to be arrested

for distributing "Counterfeit Aspirin" from a barn somewhere in New York City was found "dead under peculiar circumstances."[80] Respectable pharmacists could not afford to be associated with miscreants and criminals; all pharmacists must obey the law. The New York Retail Druggists Association, for example, stated that it "now unconditionally recognized Bayer's Aspirin patent 'until voided by a court of last resort,' and forbade any moral or financial support to members caught again buying from smugglers."[81] A benevolent Bayer did not pursue litigation if the offending druggists showed repentance. A sampling of Aspirin in New York City in June 1913 confirmed that counterfeit products were not prevalent (only 28 of 200 were adulterated). It seems that "the druggists had finally changed their behavior."[82] And Bayer, of course, still retained firm control of a product that even when competing with smugglers had brought in more than $38,000 a month.[83] The USP's eventual decision to exclude ASA from the ninth revision was neither here nor there as far as Bayer was concerned, as long as it could own the name. But the up-coming expiration of the patent cast serious doubts on just how many more years Bayer would be the owner. The AMA and the APhA had reluctantly supported Bayer's property rights as a matter of law but were still opposed to patented and trademarked drugs on principle. There was no guarantee that the name Aspirin would not become public after February 1917. The company therefore decided to review its marketing strategies.

One approach it considered was a new emphasis on the name Bayer. Although advertisements had almost always referred to "Bayer's" products, the company itself was known in the United States by various other names (Continental Color, Farbenfabriken of Elberfeld, Elberfelder); doctors and pharmacists were not altogether aware that Farbenfabriken was the source of Bayer's products. Besides, the name Farbenfabriken of Elberfeld was a tongue twister for Americans.[84] This difficulty was resolved in June 1913, with the creation of the Bayer Company, Inc., as owner of the trademarks and the Synthetic Patents Company, Inc., as owner of the patents (the majority stockholder in the latter case being Dr. Hugo Schweitzer). Both companies were legally independent of the German firm, but the head office was very much involved, receiving half of the profits from American sales.[85] Bayer, Inc., continued to report its activities to the parent company on a regular basis. The restructuring did not affect day-to-day operations, although the New York office was now in charge of Canadian markets. It is not clear what impact, if any, this had on smuggling: generic ASA remained cheaper in Canada, costing a mere thirteen cents per ounce in 1913; Bayer was still cheaper in the United States.[86]

Another marketing tactic American Bayer considered was to manufacture Aspirin in tablet form, not just as a powder. Tablets were the public's preference, and sales of Aspirin powder to tablet manufacturers had already become an important part of the company's business. At least five companies (Parke-Davis, Eli Lilly, Sharp and Dohme, J. Wyeth, and Schieffelin) bought Bayer's powder, which Bayer then allowed them to market under the name of aspirin. The fact that aspirin tablets with other companies' names on the labels were available before World War I but that Bayer Aspirin tablets were not simply added to the general confusion.[87]

Tablets were also tricky to make, and although Bayer manufactured good-quality Aspirin tablets in Germany, it had not yet done so in the United States solely because in tablet form ASA exhibited a chemical reaction that identified it as salicylic acid, a substance known to science long before Aspirin came along. It was this chemical reaction, in fact, that had lost Bayer the British patent. So in defending its U.S. patent, Bayer had made its case on the reaction's absence when its powder was tested. It had feared that a test of the tablets might result in the invalidation of the patent.[88] (Presumably, if the reaction occurred in aspirin tablets from Lilly or Wyeth, these companies' manufacturing techniques could be blamed.)

Another reason Bayer hesitated to make its own tablets was that it would be in direct competition with the tablet manufacturers to which it sold the powder—companies that had contributed to Bayer's healthy sales figures because they "had in their employ an extraordinarily large number of salesmen who visited all the retailers throughout the country." Parke-Davis was said to have 284 detailmen in the United States and 50 more outside the country. Bayer had no such sales staff. Besides, "there existed a keen competition among these manufacturers in the sale of Aspirin tablets, and prices had been lowered to such an extent that there was hardly any profit." Bayer could choose to undersell them all, which would not hurt Bayer, but it "would ruin [the other companies'] business and they would stop buying their supplies of aspirin from us. . . . This would . . . make enemies of them" and deprive Bayer of "their good will and selling power." Bayer should leave well enough alone and "abstain from market-ing Aspirin tablets."[89] So for the time being the company decided to leave tablet-making to its manufacturing customers, and before World War I, no aspirin tablet in America carried the Bayer name or logo.[90]

As an ethical firm, Bayer had always been careful not to promote its medicinal products to the public and had directed all its advertising to the medical and pharmaceutical professions. Yet if Americans indeed were consuming all the Aspirin produced by Bayer (in 1909 Bayer sold more than 686,000 ounces or about 66 million doses, a figure that does not include what was allegedly smuggled), clearly at some point the drug had become very popular with the public, more so perhaps than with physi-cians, given that neither prescription surveys nor the medical literature indicate that Aspirin was prescribed more than Phenacetin at this point. With the patent expiration looming ever closer, Bayer could not afford to ignore the implications of this popularity.

But whatever Bayer might or might not have decided to do, by the late summer of 1914 it was faced with a new emergency: the outbreak of the war in Europe. Circumstances would now conspire to set Aspirin on a new course, one in which the headache—subsumed up to this point, perhaps, in the discussion of business and other matters—would now become inex-tricably linked with this drug, influencing attitudes and treatment for the rest of the century.

7

Did the Headache
Finally Meet Its Match?

In July 1916, amid great excitement, the cargo submarine *Deutschland* slipped under the British blockade and arrived in Baltimore. It was rumored to be carrying contraband but apparently contained only mail and drug intermediates—a small load of 750 tons that nevertheless was worth at least a million dollars. This was front page news for the *New York Times* and the *New York Tribune*, and both newspapers informed their readers that the Bayer Company was among the German firms eagerly awaiting the cargo.[1] The activities of Germans in the United States had been newsworthy on several previous occasions, as rumors of espionage, sabotage, and skullduggery created bold headlines and a cloak-and-dagger atmosphere. On 17 and 18 August 1915, for example, the *New York World* ran a story that said a German agent had bought more than a million pounds of phenol from Thomas Edison's factory, where it was used for making phonograph records. The headlines tell the story: "Germany, While Seeking Embargo to Balk Allies, Secretly Arranges to Get American Arms and Supplies. Dr. Hugo Schweitzer . . . Made Deal for Phenol, Used for Explosives." Two days later Schweitzer defended his actions, telling the *World*'s readers that he had already sold the phenol to the Heyden Company to be converted to medicines, "especially the universal medicine, aspirin."[2] The story did not mention the Bayer Company, however, or that Schweitzer worked for it.

There were many Americans sympathetic to the Allied cause who were ready to find all German companies—particularly Bayer—and their representatives guilty of subterfuge, the more so as unrestricted submarine warfare took its toll and stories of atrocities in Belgium circulated.[3] Yet Thomas Reimer, in examining the allegations against both Bayer and Schweitzer, found no merit in the charges that they were involved in any of the illegal activities of which they were accused. Edison had not been tricked into the sale. Opposed to the war, he simply did not want his phenol to be made into bombs. Schweitzer did, in fact, use German government money in this transaction, but he was acting as a purchasing agent, not as a secret agent. And he was not acting for Bayer, at least not officially.[4] Whatever Bayer's German employees may or may not have been doing on behalf of the German war effort, the company was itself preoccupied with rather more mundane affairs: how to maintain control of the ASA market once the patent expired in February 1917, and how to make sure that the word *aspirin* would not become public property at the same time.

The most immediate problem for New York Bayer was the continuing scarcity of raw materials created by the blockade and embargo. But this problem also existed for its potential competitors in the ASA market in that virtually all American organic chemical production, including Bayer's, depended on German intermediates. Bayer, therefore, hoped to turn the situation to its advantage: if it used all of its own limited ASA production for the manufacture of its own Aspirin tablets (there now being no real objections to this dose form), other companies that depended on Bayer for their supplies of ASA would have to give up making ASA tablets altogether and Bayer would have the market to itself. At the very least, Bayer would still have the trade name, and its tablets labeled Bayer-Aspirin would familiarize Americans with the name while the chemical was still under patent.[5]

Not everyone in the American branch of the company agreed to this strategy. Schweitzer feared that it would make the word *aspirin* too freely available—and that the name would become public by default, regardless of what the law said. The head office had in fact suggested licensing an American firm to use Bayer's process to make what would be sold as acetylsalicylic acid tablets, so that a generic version of the drug would be on the market when the patent expired and Bayer could then argue that "the product was not known in the trade only by the name Aspirin." But it was far from certain that this plan would work. Bayer was clearly worried that

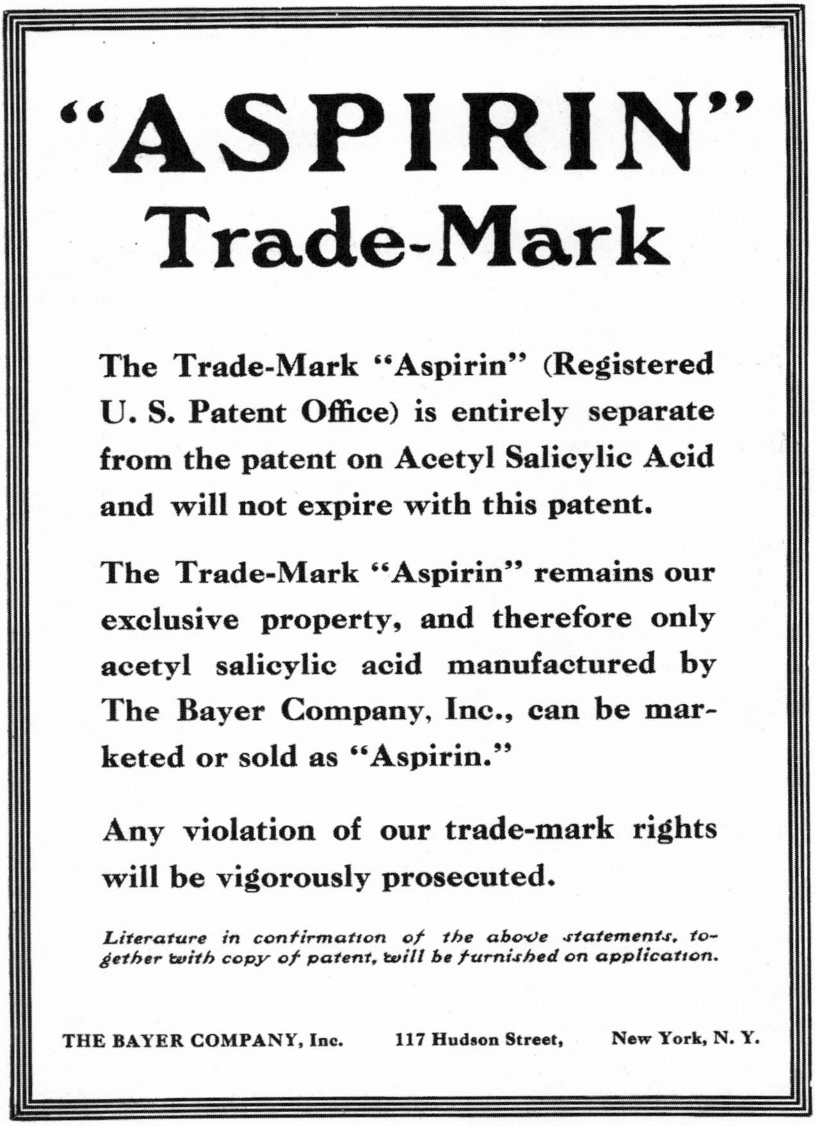

"ASPIRIN"
Trade-Mark

The Trade-Mark "Aspirin" (Registered U. S. Patent Office) is entirely separate from the patent on Acetyl Salicylic Acid and will not expire with this patent.

The Trade-Mark "Aspirin" remains our exclusive property, and therefore only acetyl salicylic acid manufactured by The Bayer Company, Inc., can be marketed or sold as "Aspirin."

Any violation of our trade-mark rights will be vigorously prosecuted.

Literature in confirmation of the above statements, together with copy of patent, will be furnished on application.

THE BAYER COMPANY, Inc.   117 Hudson Street,   New York, N. Y.

FIGURE 5. This ad appeared soon after the ASA patent expired, reminding druggists of Bayer's property rights. Unlike most other advertising, this copy appeared in the text pages, where it would not be overlooked.

From *Deutsch-Amerikanischer Apotheker-Zeitung* 38 (March 1917): 5.

the upcoming patent expiration would also mean the loss of the trade name. Furthermore, starting in about 1906 (in response to the Phenacetin problem and perhaps to the new drug label law), Bayer itself had confused the nomenclature situation by identifying Aspirin in its advertising as "the monoacetic acid ester of salicylic acid," a term no one else used and that caused physicians to indeed wonder whether ASA and Aspirin were the same thing. But Bayer's own internal memoranda and documents *always* called this chemical acetylsalicylic acid. As one drug journal declared later, Bayer's public use of the unfamiliar designation was "a dodge to keep just ahead of the law."[6] The more awkward the alternative, the more likely it was that prescribers would continue to use the term Aspirin, which Bayer was prepared to argue was its exclusive property. The Phenacetin story was a constant reminder of how tenacious Bayer could be about such matters.

At any rate, Bayer Tablets of Aspirin finally came on the market in the United States, in greater or lesser quantities according to the availability of the raw materials.[7] Tins of twelve and bottles of twenty-four or one hundred began to be advertised in medical and pharmaceutical journals, with the Bayer Cross logo stamped on each tablet and the package sporting an attractive yellow and brown design, familiar to users of Bayer products even today. (The American office, in fact, claimed to have invented the Bayer Cross.)[8] Such packages, of course, were "consumer-ready," and although Bayer's advertising at this point was still directed at pharmacists and the medical profession, the public was not entirely ignored. Some prominent ethical manufacturers in the United States (such as Parke-Davis) had already tacitly condoned self-promotion on packages because it familiarized the patient with the name of the company and made it less likely that a druggist would substitute a house brand, although direct advertising to the laity was still severely proscribed. Physicians were a profitable market all by themselves, and their growing influence on legislators and public opinion made the ethical branch of the drug industry wary of offending them.[9] Despite their many questionable practices, a significant number of ethical manufacturers simply did not wish to jeopardize what by now had become a comfortable association with the medical profession. But Bayer's fear—that despite its efforts, the courts would eventually give the term *aspirin* to the public and it would enter nomenclature limbo—demanded that the company now rethink its own position on public promotion.

There were few agreeable precedents. Lambert Pharmacal in 1914 had decided to publicly market its antiseptic liquid Listerine as a mouthwash, but because the AMA had never accepted Listerine as anything other than a nostrum, this activity did not offend professional sensibilities and merely identified the concoction by its true colors.[10] The claim that newspaper articles had been de facto advertisements for the synthetics when they were first introduced may still have held true to some extent, but Aspirin does not seem to be mentioned much in the papers, and the occasional references to other Bayer products were not always the best publicity for them. Take the case of a young man in 1906 who asked his doctor for Veronal. The doctor had never heard of this Bayer sedative and had to ask his patient how to spell the name, although he prescribed it anyway. The young man died after taking the drug. The man presumably had read about Veronal (phenobarbital) in the newspapers, although the physician apparently had not. (He was severely criticized for his ignorance.)[11]

The only justification for public advertising, according to Hugo Schweitzer, was if "a large profit was absolutely certain." Bayer, he said, had long prided itself on good relations with the American Medical Association:

We worked hand in hand and on the whole remained exempt from their attacks, while almost every other firm—such as Parke Davis & Co., Schieffelin & Co., and similar American and European manu-facturers were attacked most vehemently. If this Association were to find out that we are behind the sale of Aspirin tablets as a patent medicine, whether we do it under our own name or under that of another firm—for the Association would quickly find out who the owner was—their entire rage would be directed against us for this particular reason, because we would have turned away from them and gone over to the enemy camp. It is not to be counted out, that, if popular advertising for Aspirin is successful, the American Med-ical Association will use every means at their disposal to retaliate and hinder our sales. Because of the great influence of this Associa-tion on members of the government and legislative bodies, it could very well happen that Aspirin might be withdrawn from over-the-counter sale. If the drug is no longer useful, it also cannot be counted out that the Association could see to it that Aspirin only be sold under "narcotic orders" like morphine, and so on.[12]

Popular advertising would be very expensive, too, no less than $500,000 a year, according to Schweitzer. The problem of product substitution would remain; the term *aspirin* almost certainly would become generic. Only the name Bayer would be protected—and that was not even an American name but one belonging to a foreign, a "'Dutch' Concern." The hope that the Bayer Company would be able to convince authorities that the term *acetylsalicylic acid* belonged to the public and leave Aspirin in private hands was faint. Finally, if the war continued to affect supplies of raw materials, public advertising might create a demand that the company would be unable to meet.[13]

Schweitzer's concerns were nonetheless overruled, and a public advertising campaign was initiated, one that would be unique in the annals of proprietary medicine: "No selling talk of any kind will be used. The reader will not be urged to buy anything. The product will not be suggested as a remedy for any ailment. The uses to which it can be put will not be mentioned. The sole object of the publicity is trade-mark identification."[14] In July 1916, the first advertisements for Bayer Aspirin began to appear in major American newspapers such as the *New York Times*. In fact, the first *Times* ad appeared on 10 July 1916, the very day the *Deutschland* arrived.[15] The advertisement, at the top of page 3 in the first section, was large and informed readers that "To protect the public against spurious and adulterated Aspirin, the sole makers of the Genuine Aspirin mark every package and tablet with 'The Bayer Cross.'" There was an illustration of a bottle and a tin, as well as a tablet. By autumn, new copy appeared at least once and sometimes twice a week in the *Times*; most had illustrations of the packages with the Bayer Cross logo and "Bayer-Tablets of Aspirin" in prominent type, along with the statement that the tablets were "the monoacetic acid ester of salicylic acid." The goal was more than just trade-mark identification, however. The not-so-subtle subtext of these advertisements was the danger to individuals and their loved ones if they used anything other than Bayer. In the *Times* of 19 February 1917, for example, the copy declared that "counterfeits and substitutes may be ineffective, and even harmful. Refuse them. Protect yourself by demanding Bayer-Tablets of Aspirin." Obviously, readers were to associate Bayer with purity, efficacy, and safety.

The AMA reacted much as Schweitzer had feared. The Council on Pharmacy and Chemistry asked Bayer to respond to its objections to the overt newspaper advertising and the implicit advertising on the "vest-pocket boxes" of Aspirin tablets, but the "company's reply contained nothing to warrant the continued recognition of this product by the Council. It was accordingly directed that Aspirin-Bayer be omitted from *New and Nonofficial Remedies.*"[16]

The AMA once again urged its members to prescribe by scientific name. "Of course," added *JAMA*'s editor rather sarcastically, "for those who have been writing 'aspirin' it will be rather difficult to write 'acetylsalicylic acid,' just as a quarter of a century ago it was difficult for the physician of that day who had been using the copyright name 'antifebrin' to write 'acetanilid,' a name which nowadays is easy, even for laymen."[17]

However it might be written, it still meant only the Bayer product, at least until 27 February 1917, at which time other chemical manufacturers and tablet makers could put their own products on the market. According to the *Philadelphia Public Ledger*, the patent expiration was bringing "promises of lively times in pharmaceutical circles," with American manufacturers intending to call their product "aspirin" and Bayer promising to sue them if they did—as the Monsanto Chemical Company of St. Louis promptly found out. Even so, the drug's popularity meant that chemical shortages and litigation notwithstanding, profits were expected to be healthy.[18] By the summer of 1918, *JAMA* could list at least seven brands of ASA that conformed to the standards of its *New and Nonofficial Remedies* (*NNR*). Of these, however, only the Lehn and Fink brand called itself aspirin.[19] But there were many other tablet companies, jobbers, and manufacturers that had no interest in pleasing the AMA, were clearly targeting the public, and intended to identify their drug by the word with which most Americans were already familiar.

Bayer served notice early that it considered all such use a violation of its rights and that it would take infringers to court. A notice appearing in the February 1917 issue of the *Chicago Retail Druggists Association News* reminded readers that "any violation of our trade-mark rights will be vigorously prosecuted" (oddly, in this text the word in question is misspelled once as Asperin), but this did not prove to be much of a deterrent.[20] Lehn and Fink, for example, announced—as they had years before with phenacetin—that they would "protect against suit, by the owners of the former patent, any Druggist who sold ASPIRIN (LEHN & FINK); that we would assume all the legal burdens, expenses and responsibilities in case of suit." (They added: "We cannot, of course, undertake any responsibility—legal or otherwise—where other brands of aspirin are in question.")[21] The United Drug Company of Boston, owner of the Rexall brand name and a chain of drugstores, similarly indicated it would call their product "aspirin" at the retail level, petitioning in March for the cancellation of the trademark.[22] Later in March Bayer filed suit against the United Drug Company for infringement, intending the suit as a test case. The Detroit-based *Bulletin of Pharmacy* remarked that the case could go either way and that it would be a stormy one, but advised the trade to use the term "acetylsalicylic acid" "until the lowering clouds on the horizon have discharged some of their electricity."[23] Within a month, however, the Bayer Company had more to worry about than its patent and trade name. On 6 April 1917 the United States declared war on Germany and by August had established the office of the Alien Property Custodian (APC), whose goal was to track down and confiscate any and all German-owned property, both physical and intellectual, no matter how well disguised as American. Bayer was one of the principal targets.[24]

On the surface at least, there was a good case against Bayer. Hugo Schweitzer, the company's chief chemist and owner of most of the patents (as owner of Synthetic Patents, Inc.), was a naturalized American, but he had been vociferously pro-German before the United States entered the war, having written several pamphlets that condemned Great Britain and encouraged American neutrality; he was also implicated in the Great Phenol Plot of 1915. But because he died of pneumonia in December 1917, he was never interrogated, and the extent of his involvement was never fully explored. The *New York Times* reported his death without comment on 24 December and noted a week later that a memorial service was scheduled for the Chemical Club in January. At the last minute, however, the service was "emphatically forbidden" by the board of trustees of the Chemical Club, although fifty people showed up anyway.[25] Rumors questioning Schweitzer's loyalty had apparently started to circulate. It was later said that he had been a German spy, the "chief cook and bottle washer of the German Government in this country," one of the leaders of the supposedly 250,000 German agents in the United States.[26] (If such an assemblage ever did exist, however, it was hopelessly inept.)[27] Nonetheless, Schweitzer had been in charge of a large amount of German government money, possibly to facilitate espionage and sabotage, but more likely to aid in a propaganda campaign to counteract the British before America entered the war.[28] In fact, as Thomas Reimer has shown, most of the allegations against Schweitzer (and Bayer) were made up after the war to justify the government's otherwise dubiously legal confiscation of German property.[29] The property, of course, was worth millions.

At first, the reorganization of Bayer in 1913 as a New York corporation hid the fact that the real owners of the company were in Germany, but by the spring of 1918, the APC had seized the company's property and assets, its managers had been interned, and it was being run by government appointees, who nonetheless seem to have been dedicated to keeping the firm as profitable as ever, treating Aspirin, for instance, just as the German owners had, much to the annoyance of some patriotic Americans. ("Surely," said a leading engineering periodical, "the Custodian would not care, even in a trustee capacity, to continue in a misleading campaign whose sole purpose is the perpetuation of a monopoly hitherto enjoyed under full patent protection.")[30] But despite advertising in both the public and trade press that "ASPIRIN has been made in the United States Since 1904" and that the Bayer Company was indeed "100% American," supervised by "American Officers and Directors," Americans were not sure how remote the Germans actually were from American Bayer's operations.[31] Suspecting that property and profits might be returned to Germany after the war, many druggists wrote to the government that they "would not be a party to the sale of a penny's worth of [Bayer's] products."[32] "We are 100% AMERICANS in this firm, and will NOT purchase any product that is not strictly PRO-ALLY in every respect."[33] Even the National Association of Retail Druggists was unsure of Bayer's real status and stated its disdain for "all enterprises that emanate from Germany."[34]

Physicians, too, expressed similar sentiments. An Illinois doctor objected not only to the high price Americans had always had to pay for Aspirin but said that this now amounted to an indirect tax that was assisting Germany's attempts "to exterminate the rest of humanity."[35] In April 1918, a Dr. John Bowker of Massachusetts reminded the APC that in an earlier letter he had stated his "hope that [the Bayer Company's] money might no longer go to Germany to be *turned into bullets to kill our boys*." Even though the APC had taken over the company, he was still fearful: "if the same chemists, technicians etc. are to be retained, we have no guarantee that their personal funds will not reach Germany, sooner or later." That this had already happened, he had "absolute knowledge." He knew, for example, that German reservists worked for the company, that one employee

> is guilty of the lowest of crimes and that another is now at Fort
> Oglethorpe, detained as a spy. I protest earnestly against our Gov-
> ernment being a partner to any deal that allows such characters to
> take our money while our lads are *shedding their blood in France.*
> Reflect for a moment, that while we scrimp to buy bonds to *defend*
> us, we pay money to German firms to destroy us?[36]

Investigators did look into these and other allegations but were generally convinced that "the German influence in the Company [was] substantially eliminated as to the employees."[37] Correspondents were also told that Bayer's profits bought Liberty Bonds but that what happened to the company and its assets after the war was up to Congress.[38]

The confusion about whether Bayer was still German arose in part from the fact that other than making patriotic statements in their adver-tising, the Americans who ran Bayer on behalf of the APC made no obvious changes in the Aspirin campaign and tried to preserve Bayer's control of the trade name with as much enthusiasm as the original owners. The infringement suit against the United Drug Company was not dropped; public advertisements continued to tell Americans "that for their 'protec-tion' they should buy the product of the Bayer Company, and thus secure the 'genuine' and avoid 'imitations' and 'substitutes'" which 'may prove ineffective and harmful.'" Bayer Aspirin was twice as expensive as other brands.[39] A West Virginia druggist even reported that a Bayer salesman had told him, "our Company does not recognize the various other brands you handle as Aspirin at all." The salesman had said that because of the federal government's involvement, if the druggist continued to display non-Bayer ASA as aspirin, "you might some day have a government man step in and cause you some trouble."[40]

There was also a good deal of negative publicity in the public arena. "Will you kindly write me," inquired L. Ruby Reid, a Red Cross worker from

North Carolina, in a letter to the Department of Justice, "if the Government has had an analysis of Asperin [*sic*] tablets and found any germs in them? There are 'whispers' to this effect in my community, especially in regard to the Bayer brand."[41] Although some Bayer newspaper advertisements, like their trade journal counterparts, expressed a patriotic fervor ("100% American," adorned with eagles, and so on), Aspirin's association with the enemy seems to have been quite well known to the general public.[42] Mrs. Reid was concerned that the poison stories were German propaganda, designed to frighten people away from a drug that was "so effective in helping prevent the influenza," which was a raging pandemic in late 1918. There was an even larger segment of the population, on the other hand, that suspected Bayer Aspirin tablets were "the reason for the rapid spread of the 'flu.'"[43] One correspondent had heard that the government "had secured absolute proof that the Chief Chemist of the Bayer, Inc. had been putting dangerous drugs in aspirin tablets," which accounted for the "rapid spread of Influenza at Camp Devens."[44] "One hears rumors," noted a Philadelphia man, "that the Bayer Aspirin is infected and causes disease; and one is naturally suspicious of any medicinal preparation put out by houses with German names."[45] A Baltimore woman said her doctor told her "that [aspirin] was a very dangerous drug to take." She also noticed "that the aspirin in bulk [was] more grey and chalky looking than it used to be." Was it true that the drug was "in German hands"?[46] There were even newspaper stories to give credence to the rumors; all over the country people were reported to be returning or destroying their Bayer tablets, fearing it was contaminated with the Spanish influenza.

Some members of the public also suspected that Aspirin advertisements were "conveying information to the enemy" via code numbers that appeared in the copy, a prospect that at least one military intelligence officer viewed with "grave suspicion."[47] Government agents duly investigated the stories of poisoned drugs and encoded advertisements but concluded there was nothing substantive in either case.[48]

Despite the bad publicity, hostile pharmacists, and difficulties in obtaining the chemicals necessary for the production of Aspirin, in one four-month period in 1918 Bayer managed to sell more than $2.2 million worth of goods and make a comfortable profit. The records did not single out Aspirin sales, but it is not unreasonable to assume that the drug accounted for a large percentage of this figure, as it had before the war.[49] The deputy alien property custodian, Francis Garvan, believed that Bayer attracted so much attention from prospective purchasers of the property because "their profits on aspirin are something very, very high. I think the real asset of that business was the aspirin business."[50] But when the APC announced in late 1918 that Bayer Company, Inc., would be put on the auction block, more than just large drug companies and chemical manufacturers were interested. An Iowa doctor asked "how much stock would a person have to buy to get a little," and a Minnesota druggist wrote to Bayer that "when the stock . . . is put on sale I want a few shares, if it would be possible." Someone at Bayer scribbled "me too" on the letter.[51]

The auction took place on Thursday, 12 December 1918. The high bid of $5.3 million came from Sterling Products, of Wheeling, West Virginia, a company that up to this point had been known only for its vigorous promotion of nostrums, acting as a holding company for a number of well-known but "unethical" patent medicines. Selling the dyestuffs part of the concern to Grasselli Chemical Company, Sterling retained Bayer Company, Inc., solely to manufacture and market Aspirin and Aspirin compounds, and created the Winthrop Chemical Company to handle Bayer's ethical products. Although the company in Germany (now located in Leverkusen) was most unhappy with this situation and in fact managed to negotiate a number of agreements with the Americans that involved trademarks, patent rights, trade secrets, new German products, and the South American and Canadian markets, Sterling was adamant that Bayer Aspirin in the United States would remain under American control.[52]

Whatever Sterling gained from its association with German Bayer, its advertising campaign for Bayer Tablets of Aspirin was far more extensive than the German company had ever considered—with a budget of one million dollars—although at first the differences were not particularly noticeable. The newspaper campaign continued much as before, emphasizing the purity of Bayer Aspirin and the hazards of all the non-Bayer imitations. On Monday, 6 January 1919, for example, a large advertisement on the second page of the *New York Times* reproduced in facsimile a newspaper article with the headline "Drug Maker Arrested in Aspirin Case," describing the activities of a Brooklyn man who at the time of his arrest had in his possession nearly 400,000 "Aspirin" tablets made of talcum powder. Officials estimated that he sold about half a million such tablets every month, with dire consequences for public health. "Now you know why you must Look for the Bayer Cross," warned the Bayer headline. Although this copy was very likely placed by the pre-Sterling managers and seems to have referred to one of the pre-war counterfeit scandals, the new owners retained this alarmed tone for many subsequent advertisements, once again rousing the ire of pharmacists, who resented the implication that their profession was still being accused of passing bogus drugs to the public, either from greed or ignorance, and who were not entirely convinced even yet that German Bayer was not behind it all. The *American Journal of Pharmacy* expressed great displeasure that the American owners had "committed the error of continuing the Hun method of advertising."[53] Canadian pharmacists were so upset with Sterling-Bayer that they ejected the company's representative from their 1919 annual convention, believing that "German propaganda was still in operation in Canada" and vowing to "unite against any German trade aggression."[54]

Faced with such attitudes, the new Bayer (Sterling) therefore changed its strategy, hoping to mollify the druggists and make them think of themselves as partners, in a sense, in a profitable American enterprise. (In order to buy Bayer in the first place, Sterling had had to prove to the APC that all company officers were American citizens and that they had no business ties to Germany.) The firm therefore withdrew the offending advertisements; it guaranteed to take back unsold stock for cash and provided free window and counter displays, tips on sales techniques, and handsome profit margins. Then, to help attract customers, the company spent its million dollar advertising budget on a national promotional campaign in North American newspapers and magazines that drew on Sterling's own experience as a preeminent nostrum marketer.

When Sterling bid for the German company in 1918, the American firm was less than twenty years old but owned a number of popular remedies, including Cascarets Candy Cathartic, Fletcher's Castoria, California Syrup of Figs, Dr. James' Headache Powders, and Dodson's Liver Tone. From the first, "advertising was embraced as a guiding principle," and by about 1914, the company had respectable annual profits in the neighborhood of $800,000.[55]

Pre-war Sterling appears to have adopted an advertising policy of the type that the AMA found particularly offensive but that was evidently successful. Compositors setting up advertisements for Dr. James' Headache Powders, for example, were instructed to "add to, or take from, any word or letter you see fit, necessary to make copy appear like regular news; but do not change the sense of reading." The sense, of course, was that these powders were quick to act, effective, and endorsed by millions.[56] In other cases, compositors were asked to set the copy in the regular typeface of their newspaper; they were also informed that "the word advertisement, abbreviation thereof or other advertisement marks, will not be allowed" to appear in or near the copy. When newspapers advertised several of Sterling's products, some of which were in competition with one another, the papers were told to "never permit any two of our advertisements to appear adjoining one another." They must always be put "on different parts of the page or different pages of your paper." A proof for California Syrup of Figs (a laxative) was in fact stamped with a notice that "no credit [would] be allowed for this advertising when placed on same page with CASTORIA copy."[57] Castoria, another Sterling product, was a laxative intended for children, and in promoting it, Sterling did not neglect another hallmark of nostrum advertising: to inform the consumer of the uses to which the product could be put and to suggest any number of dire consequences should a symptom be ignored. "Save the Babies!" cried a Castoria ad in the *Baltimore Sun* in 1906. Surely no mother would let a constipated child continue to suffer after such an appeal.[58]

Despite having many of the attributes of the most offensive patent medicine manufacturers, Sterling's pre-Bayer products acquired a certain amount of respect. The most popular of them did not contain narcotics or much alcohol and were no worse than anything else on the market. In fact, William Weiss, one of Sterling's founders, in 1915 had proposed a resolution for the Proprietary Association of America to consider. It condemned nostrums that claimed unreasonable cures (especially for serious diseases), approved of the Harrison Narcotic Act, and requested that the association's members submit their packages and literature for in-house inspection.[59]

With Bayer Aspirin there was no doubt as to the product's scientific and medical credentials, and Sterling did not muddy the waters by associating its newest acquisition with its less prestigious products. Newspaper advertisements for Cascarets and Danderine that appeared in the same issue as advertisements for Aspirin, for example, did not inform readers that all these items were handled by the same company. The AMA, however, was well aware of the new owners: "By half-truths and inferential falsehoods, the public has been led to believe that the only genuine aspirin on the market is the one put out under the Bayer name. The facts are, of course, that the aspirin of any reputable firm is just as good as the aspirin put out by the makers of Livertone, Danderine and Cascarets."[60]

When Sterling took over Aspirin, the newspaper advertising already in place had deliberately avoided naming the ailments for which Aspirin might be used—an obvious contrast with other proprietary promotions and in keeping with the virtuous attitude that German Bayer had assumed. Sterling maintained the same style for several years, at least in the advertisements intended for the *New York Times* and other prestigious papers. Nonetheless, there is evidence that in less-distinguished publications less restraint was required, as when a pseudo-news piece appeared on the front page of the *Cleveland Gazette* (an African-American weekly), on 15 November 1919, with the headline "Take Aspirin with Water"—immediately, and rather jarringly, below the paper's huge main headline about a horrific lynching in Arkansas. Such an advertisement may also have been the sort referred to by a doctor who sent *JAMA* a news clipping of a "syndicated article" whose writer, he suspected, was in the "pay of the Bayer people . . . helping them to put across their advertising campaign."[61]

These advertisements now contained indications for use of the drug: "Take Aspirin. For headache, neuralgia, toothache, aching gums, earache, rheumatism, sciatica, gout, neuritis, colds, grippe, influenzal colds, stiff neck, distress, lame back, lumbago, joint pains. Pain! Pain!" An enormous variety of advertisements seems to have been developed: "Oh! Such Relief!" "Like Magic Touch!" "Whole Day Saved!" "Mercy's Gift." "The servant of mercy for the pain stricken!" "One of the Great Blessings of Life." Indeed, in an enthusiastic text sent to the nation's druggists some time in 1919, Sterling proclaimed, "For the first time in pharmaceutical history the uses and dosage of Bayer Tablets of Aspirin are being advertised." Pain, especially headache pain, was prominently listed as succumbing to Aspirin's power. "This is part of the effective million dollar campaign for this wonderful product now in full swing. The smashing every day drive through newspapers everywhere is increasing demand to a remarkable degree."[62] Sterling's enormous profits demonstrated that the purchase price had been entirely realistic: in 1919 alone the company cleared more than two million dollars. Millions of Americans using Aspirin for pain—and especially for headache pain—were the principal reason.

The present association of aspirin and headaches is so entrenched in American culture that it might seem that this relationship must have existed from the time the drug was introduced in 1899, but Bayer first presented the drug as an ethical specific for the treatment of rheumatic afflictions. It first made a name for itself as an excellent antirheumatic remedy. According to one Harvard-educated physician,

> aspirin was . . . very popular from the start. Old gentlemen told other old gentlemen of the favorable effect of aspirin on their rheumatism or gouty pains. For a time, in Boston, it was known as the Somerset Club remedy. For in the Somerset Club, the old gentlemen swapped tales of the efficiency of this new wonder drug.[63]

Aspirin was, however, a wonder drug that neither Bayer nor the medical profession considered to be competitive with Phenacetin or the other antipyretic analgesics. Bayer's advertisements identified Aspirin as "an agreeable and efficient substitute for the salicylates" or "the best antirheumatic," whereas Phenacetin was described as "the safest and most effective antipyretic and analgesic." In the hundreds of articles that were published worldwide in the first decade of Aspirin's existence, it is rare to find one championing the drug as a general pain or headache remedy unless the pain or headache had a rheumatic cause.[64] In the pre-war years, evidence in fact suggests that American doctors were not as excited about Aspirin as they had been about the earlier coal tar drugs. A Milwaukee druggist's records indicate he filled only three prescriptions for Aspirin from 1902 through 1904, two of them from the same doctor.[65] A survey in 1909 found that for every 10,000 prescriptions, 136 were for Aspirin whereas 227 were for Phenacetin; 92.5 were for salicylic acid.[66] The *New York Times*, which had had a good deal to say about the earlier drugs, scarcely mentioned Aspirin before World War I.

On the surface, therefore, the increasing use of the drug as a household analgesic appears to have been the result of Sterling's tireless promotion, "a remarkable example of what propaganda can accomplish."[67] Yet although there is no doubt that Sterling's campaign did increase sales, the advertising did not create the association between Aspirin and the headache in the public mind. That association was already well established. By 1906, Farbenfabriken Bayer in Germany reported that Aspirin was "the most used and beloved medicine we manufacture . . . [whose] notable analgesic effect on all sorts of conditions . . . [has made it] 'a household remedy in the true sense of the word.'"[68] By 1913, British authors were reporting that "aspirin [was] probably more frequently employed than any other medicinal substance."[69] Given that headaches were more common than acute rheumatism, headaches were very likely responsible for this statistic. We have already noted that Aspirin replaced Phenacetin as American Bayer's best seller and must assume that in America, too, rheumatic patients were not the only reason for this success, although many patients who were prescribed Aspirin for their inflamed joints undoubtedly continued to use it for other kinds of pain.

In the American context, at least, the 1906 Pure Food and Drug Act may also have contributed to Aspirin's popularity. Acetylsalicylic acid did not have any of the side effects of the aniline derivatives and seemed to be virtually risk free (except for occasional allergic or salicylate-related reactions), so doctors may have recommended it as a painkiller because of its relative safety. Anecdotal evidence supports this possibility. Dr. Roger Lee, who entered Harvard medical school in 1901, remembered that it was quite common to hear a doctor on the telephone say to a patent with a headache: "Of course, you have some aspirin in the house. Take one tablet now and two at bedtime and if you are not better in the morning, call me."[70] An Atlanta doctor—who preferred acetanilid—in 1911 criticized his colleagues for being too ready to treat headaches with a "dose of physic and a little aspirin."[71] A British physician had found Aspirin serviceable in "severe headache occurring as the result of over-work or over-anxiety" but added that this was most effective in the presence of a "gouty diathesis," reiterating the rheumatic connection.[72] The AMA itself recognized and lamented that Aspirin was a common headache treatment when it deleted Bayer's product from the *NNR* in 1917. This is the only symptom mentioned by name in the report.[73] On the whole, however, ASA as a headache remedy did not enter the medical literature. Long after Aspirin's debut, many

physicians who wished to treat headaches with a synthetic drug still preferred Phenacetin.[74] In fact, even before the AMA considered deleting
Aspirin because of Bayer's advertising campaign, and several years before
Sterling was involved, the *NNR* had noted the "promiscuous use of acetylsalicylic acid (aspirin) by the laity, especially for the relief of headache."[75]
So if physicians were not entirely responsible for this, we must conclude
that it was the public that identified and exploited Aspirin as a headache
remedy—in such numbers that Sterling was more than willing to pay millions of dollars for the property in 1918.

Sterling was unable, however, to retain control of the name for which
it had paid so much. At the outbreak of the war in Europe, British courts
had declared that the word *aspirin* was free for anyone to use as a synonym
for ASA.[76] The French, whose laws had never tolerated drug monopolies of
any kind, apparently had been using *aspirine* as a generic from the first,
ignoring any protests from Bayer. In the United States, where Bayer had few
friends, and where American chemical manufacturers were poised to compete with the German products as soon as it was legal to do so (if not
before), it was inevitable that the trade name would become public.[77] Yet it
was not a straight path to this result. In March 1919, two years after filing,
the United Drug Company's petition for cancellation of the trademark was
granted. The examiner of interferences of the United States Patent Office
declared that the word *aspirin* was now available for public use because it
was the only name by which the drug had ever been known; moreover,
Bayer had maintained its hold on the word by fraudulent means.[78] Sterling,
however, continued its efforts to retain its "common-law right to the trade-
mark" and did not let the case drop.[79] It dragged on for another two years
until finally, in April 1921, Judge Learned Hand decided that as far as the
public was concerned, *aspirin* was indeed a generic name and that a customer who used this word could be sold any manufacturer's ASA. A physician, on the other hand, who prescribed "aspirin" was presumed to know
the difference between this and ASA, and pharmacists were therefore obligated to supply the Bayer product in this case. At the wholesale level, too,
the trade was now to restrict the term Aspirin to Bayer products and use
acetylsalicylic acid for other brands.[80] This decision had virtually no effect
on actual practice, however; druggists and doctors alike ignored it, and
aspirin became a de facto generic in the United States, although the AMA

continued to advise its members to use acetylsalicylic acid in prescriptions to avoid any possible benefit to either Sterling or German Bayer.[81]

The loss of the trade name was a serious blow to Sterling. "Ownership of the Bayer cross still gave Bayer [i.e., Sterling] a powerful competitive advantage, but nothing compared to what control of 'aspirin' would have."[82] Even before the end of the war, advertisements for other brands of aspirin had appeared in the trade press; through the 1920s and 1930s, hundreds of jobbers, suppliers, tablet companies, chain stores, individual drugstores, department stores, and other vendors marketed their own lines. Some, like Smith, Kline and French's Red Band brand, possessed colorful and attractive packages.[83] Others, like Preston, mimicked Bayer's labels and bottle shapes. But most brands were confined to local or regional markets. Only Bayer was truly national, aggressively and imaginatively advertised across the country to pharmacists and the public (but not to physicians). By 1931 many "retail druggists [bought] Bayer's aspirin as often as three times a week" because it was so much in demand.[84] By 1934, 4,817 newspapers sported a distinctive Bayer Aspirin advertisement on a regular basis, as did many of the major magazines.[85] In that same year, Bayer sponsored a program of popular music heard on seventy-five NBC radio stations and paid $750,000 per year for radio spots.[86] And though it was far more expensive than generic brands (in 1936 an Albuquerque drugstore offered one hundred tablets of Bayer for fifty-nine cents, regularly seventy-five, but a house brand for a mere thirteen cents),[87] Bayer nonetheless retained a sizeable share of the ASA market—especially the impulse buyer. According to a drug trade report in March 1935, there were only "one or two leading sellers" that could make a profit from the sale of twelve-tablet tins.[88] There is little doubt that one of these was Bayer Aspirin.

There is also little doubt that in advertising its own product, Bayer had made the word *aspirin* in general better known to the public at large and thereby lost some of its potential customers to the cheaper brands.[89] Whether consuming Bayer or another brand, however, Americans swallowed a prodigious quantity of this drug. A trade paper reported that sales in 1937 were 25 percent higher than in 1936, "a growth . . . [that was] little short of amazing," amounting to 5,143,672 pounds of aspirin or 7,201,140,800 tablets. At two tablets per dose, the journal estimated that

3,600,570,400 headaches had been cured.[90] Perhaps headaches had finally met their match.

Even so, acetanilid- and phenacetin-based headache powders and tablets were still available and popular, despite the alleged dangers of circulatory collapse and addiction.[91] One longtime headache sufferer who was also a physician said he had found Antikamnia and Pyramidon better than anything else for his own headaches and eventually settled on a combination of acetanilid, monobromate of camphor, and caffeine citrate. He never left home without it, but he does not appear to have tried to market it, evidently being the sort of doctor who liked to share his knowledge gratis.[92] A Minnesota dentist, on the other hand, having devised a recipe that was useful in his dental practice, began to sell it as An-A-Cin about 1915, although by the mid-1920s the brand had been bought by more experienced marketers, who began to advertise it nationally as a general pain and headache remedy.

Like the older proprietaries, Anacin consisted of several ingredients, usually acetphenetidin and caffeine, along with quinine sulphate and perhaps ASA (or perhaps not, according to whim; no law required that ASA be listed). Like the pre-1906 drugs, Anacin was not always candid about its ingredients. In 1929 the manufacturers were fined for misbranding because "acetphenetidin" was printed on the package in letters too small to read.[93] Interestingly, in 1930 the Anacin concern was bought by American Home Products, an umbrella company established by one of Sterling's founders as a sister organization. Anacin and Bayer Aspirin thus became cousins even as they remained rivals.[94] Nevertheless, Anacin remained fairly successful, as did a few other nationally advertised headache treatments such as Bromo-Seltzer and Alka-Seltzer, which targeted sick headaches—no hangovers, of course, during Prohibition.[95] Some, such as BC Headache Powders, became regional favorites. All, however, harked back to the older style of proprietary remedy in that they were mixtures rather than single substances and were coy about their contents, which they could change without notice.[96] They were also on the AMA's list of undesirable proprietaries, derided in *JAMA*, forbidden entry to the *NNR*, and disparaged as epitomes of fraud and greed.

Aspirin, on the other hand, had always been considered reasonably safe as well as effective. Its ubiquity as a headache remedy, however, was of some concern to a medical profession that still saw domestic treatment as a threat to professional authority and was unhappy that such an important medicine had become so accessible. But Bayer's decision in 1916 to advertise Aspirin to the public had effectively demolished any hopes that physicians would ever really control the product as a prescription drug. Federal legislation, moreover, did not deal with drug advertising, only with labels, and in any case did not include ASA.[97] Aspirin in fact had simply reinforced and improved on the long-cherished American right to treat one's headache with the best remedies available, whether or not a doctor approved. Manufacturers were only too happy to oblige.

In the 1920s the AMA founded a monthly magazine, *Hygeia*, in an effort to educate the public on prevention and public health measures. The publication emphasized the need for medical supervision of all headaches and stressed that even the omnipresent aspirin should only be "taken under the direction of a competent physician."[98] *Hygeia* never recommended self-treatment, even drugless regimens, because all headaches required an accurate diagnosis.[99] Yet aspirin, at any rate, proved difficult to demonize.[100] Did the AMA think that it "somehow mysteriously lost [its] therapeutic efficacy when [it] began to advertise directly to laymen"? asked one commentator.[101] Perhaps not, although its attractions could nevertheless lead to overuse and to inappropriate use.[102] But because negative reports about aspirin were rare, even *Hygeia* had to admit that "the indiscriminate use of [the drug] has been rather free from fatalities" and "that [aspirin] has its good points."[103] Moreover, despite the position in *Hygeia*, the AMA in the post–World War I period does not appear to have considered home treatment with aspirin to be the same sort of problem that home treatment with acetanilid or phenacetin had been. Although lay readers of *Hygeia* were told that aspirin was not harmless and that it could depress the heart and affect the blood, professional readers of *JAMA* were told that fears of cardiac involvement were "typical misinformation"; aspirin did indeed have some important side effects, but depression of the heart was not one of them.[104] Gastric distress was quite common, sometimes severe, but when a Texas physician inquired about the potential dangers of taking forty to ninety grains of aspirin a day, the reply mentioned nephritis, tinnitus, and skin rashes, not stomach upset or bleeding.[105]

Indeed, it was not the medical profession but consumer advocates who tried to raise the alarm about ASA, demanding that a law be passed requiring its presence be listed on medication labels. Arthur Kallet and F. J. Schlink, two latter-day muckrakers, pointed out that idiosyncrasy to aspirin was fairly common, which put at risk all those persons who took a product although ignorant of its contents.[106] In general, however, aspirin did not generate much consternation. When the newly founded Consumers Union published its first *Reports* in May 1936, it included an article on Alka-Seltzer (which was mostly ASA and sodium bicarbonate but never advertised as such) by a physician who noted that aspirin had a "limited but respectable place" in medicine if the drug was not abused. He accused the Alka-Seltzer company of deception not because it was ignoring hazards but because it pretended its product was something grander than it really was.[107] The August issue of *Reports* had a much more hard-hitting exposé of dangerous drugs and cosmetics, some of which were "the most heavily advertised, most widely-used products in the drug market." In fact, "the largest group in the Blacklist is the headache and pain cures, among which are . . . *Anacin Tablets*, *B.C.* [powders, and] *Bromo-Seltzer*. . . . All these products contain one or more ingredients which have caused cases of fatal poisoning . . . acetanilid, acetphenetidin, antipyrin, and aspirin." The report goes on to say, however, that aspirin is "probably the least injurious," could be used "safely in moderate amounts," was "probably the safest" of all the painkillers, and was "perhaps the only one which should be used without medical advice."[108]

Because the most prominent brand of aspirin, Bayer, was not guilty of hiding secret ingredients, *Reports* never accused the company of the same iniquities suspected of other manufacturers. But Bayer was not without sin. The painkiller industry had apparently reached the saturation point with respect to headaches. Drug makers needed a new ailment to address, and the common cold became the target. Bayer advertisements led the way in making sweeping claims for the value of taking not just two but perhaps a dozen tablets, which could be swallowed or gargled to ward off sore throats, sniffles, congestion, and—yes—headaches, or even to cure a cold outright.[109] Yet *Reports*'s concern in this case was that the money spent for an effect "entirely without foundation" was utterly wasted; because aspirin was largely harmless, only people with sensitivities to the drug were at risk.[110]

The Food and Drug Act of 1906 had proven inadequate to the task of controlling deceptive, misleading, or fraudulent advertising. Not until the New Deal administration in 1933 did a proposal to revise the law appear before Congress. This bill was largely an effort of the Food and Drug Administration (FDA, which was newly created out of the Bureau of Chemistry in 1930) to enlarge its own scope, to clarify the chain of command and bureaucratic jurisdictions, as well as to give the federal government more teeth with respect to consumer protection, including provisions about advertising.[111] The AMA was of course interested, although it was ambivalent about how much support to give to "the extension of federal authority over the nation's health and medical problems." It nevertheless "championed the idea of stronger federal power for curbing many public health abuses."[112]

For various reasons, however, the legislation stalled. Drug makers found much to complain about and "worked behind the scenes to water down the bill."[113] The public (consumers' groups notwithstanding) was not particularly interested, and there was no shocked outrage at what drug companies were doing until 1937, when the Massengill Company of Bristol, Tennessee, wishing to provide its southern customers with a liquid version of sulfanilamide, a new wonder drug from Germany, used diethylene glycol as a solvent.[114] Its Elixir Sulfanilamide, however, ended up killing more than one hundred people, all of them painfully, many of them children. The solvent the company had used was highly toxic. Yet the only law it had broken was the federal label law. By definition, an elixir must contain alcohol, which the Massengill product did not. The only legal punishment was a fine for misbranding.[115] This tragedy highlighted the inadequacies of current law, resulted in a public outcry, and prompted the passage of the Food, Drug, and Cosmetic Act of 1938.

Although this legislation was less comprehensive than its original sponsors had wanted, it did introduce some significant changes that were intended to make self-treatment safer and allow consumers to make wise choices.[116] Among other things, new drugs now had to be proven safe. (Existing drugs were largely presumed to have already demonstrated this.) Drugs, old or new, that could not be taken safely under any circumstances were banned. Active ingredients, dosages, contraindications, warnings regarding prolonged use, and so forth must appear on the label, but no misleading or fraudulent claims were permitted. And the definition of fraud was now such that it would be easier to prosecute. Medications were also to be accompanied by adequate instructions for use. If harm came to a patient despite following these instructions, the manufacturer could be found liable. To avoid that possibility, the drug company might choose to identify its product as one to be taken only on the advice of a physician (that is, by prescription), in which case it was up to the doctor to advise the patient of doses and dangers. To spare themselves a great deal of inconvenience, many drug firms began to restrict some of their products to "prescription-only," a trend that the FDA approved and encouraged, even though this was not the original intent of the law. It also produced a great deal of confusion because some manufacturers restricted a particular drug while other firms did not, and some patients obtained a drug by prescription one week but bought a legally labeled over-the-counter version of it the next. Nor did the creation of a prescription-only category even have the support of the AMA because the organization was angry that the power to decide which drugs belonged in which group was being given to the pharmaceutical industry, not the medical profession. At any rate, the FDA's interpretation of the 1938 act meant an unprecedented restriction on the traditional right to self-treatment, "a stunning change in the way drugs were to be sold."[117]

For the painkillers already in existence, however, other than requiring them to list their ingredients, the new regulations had little impact. All of them remained available over the counter. In fact, the legislation did not even cover the proprietary activity that most offended consumer and medical watchdogs—outrageous advertising. A bureaucratic squabble between the FDA and the Federal Trade Commission (FTC) resulted in the Wheeler-Lea Act of 1938, which gave responsibility for the supervision of drug advertising to the FTC. This legislation, in which the label laws did not apply, "had been designed in part . . . to prevent the Food and Drug Administration from gaining control of advertising," and although it made false or misleading advertising punishable by fine or imprisonment, it could only be invoked after the offending advertisement had been published.[118] What constituted false or misleading advertising was determined after the damage had been done. Bayer Aspirin and its competitors were therefore reasonably safe from prosecution and continued their imaginative efforts to attract customers in an ever-more-competitive environment.[119] But the headache remained the bedrock of their existence.

Of course, there were other approaches to headache relief besides taking a painkiller, as doctors were still anxious to point out: "He who depends on drug relief for headache is his own worst enemy. . . . A headache can't be cured by the simple expedient of using a drug to smash the nerves into a state of insensibility. The only sensible way is to make an intelligent effort to find the cause, and remove it."[120] A "mistreated stomach" was the usual culprit, and because most headaches went away by themselves anyway, there was nothing to be gained by taking an analgesic. In recurrent headaches, on the other hand, a more serious situation might be developing, requiring the practitioner "to form an estimate of the constitutional equipment of the individual, of his habits of mind and emotion, together with the circumstances that play upon them, and also of his physical condition and external environment."[121] In other words, if a headache was to be treated appropriately, it still required a physician's careful, educated evaluation, not the patient's amateur diagnosis, just as it had a hundred years earlier. But did the medical profession in fact have anything beyond aspirin to offer? Had science, which had done so much for other areas of medicine, discovered anything else to help the men and women for whom even Bayer or Anacin did not work?

8

The Headache in
the Twentieth Century

Visitors to the World's Fair in Chicago in 1933 flocked to one particular pavilion in such numbers "that it became one of the most popular exhibits at the exposition."[1] In addition to a marvelous "transparent man" made of plastic with organs that could light up, fairgoers also gazed at replicas of old pharmacies, dioramas depicting pre-anesthetic surgery, enlarged photographs of blood cells and disease bacteria, and charts and graphs comparing modern death rates with those of yore. The theme was "a century of progress," "the golden age of discovery in medicine," and although "it was a surprise [to the organizers] that the public interest in the exhibit was so great," they should not have been so naive. In the previous fifty years alone, well within the lifetime of many visitors and coincident with the careers of the antipyretic analgesics, medical science and the medical profession had changed drastically. The World's Fair proudly highlighted their accomplishments.

In that half century, the germ theory of disease and prophylactic inoculation had become accepted and validated. In the 1890s, x-ray technology began to revolutionize diagnostic procedures. Diphtheria antitoxin saved thousands of children from a horrible death. The roles of insects and other arthropods in transmitting diseases such as Texas cattle fever, malaria, plague, and yellow fever were demonstrated. Useful new concepts of immunity were being developed. After the turn of the century, vitamins were identified, and nutritional disorders were better understood. Tests for the presence of disease organisms (syphilis, tuberculosis, diphtheria) made early diagnosis possible and interventions more successful. Paul Ehrlich created the first "magic bullet"—a drug that specifically targeted one of those organisms. The discovery of insulin in the 1920s lifted the death sentence from diabetics. A vaccine for tuberculosis was invented, and an antitoxin for scarlet fever. In the 1930s, the first crude electron microscopes could detect viruses. Soon after the Fair ended, the Bayer section of IG Farben in Germany introduced the sulfanilamide drug Prontosil, a foretaste of the antibiotics. In these five decades, new anesthetics and operative and postoperative techniques made surgery safer (and fashionable: tonsillectomies became almost routine).[2]

By the early 1930s, the American medical profession, too, had largely become the educated, science-trained profession that orthodoxy had longed wanted. Doctors—including a growing number of women—now had to undergo rigorous training as undergraduates in schools with stricter admissions standards and a comprehensive curriculum predicated upon basic sciences. They did further training as interns and residents before practicing on their own and could not practice at all unless duly examined and licensed by the proper, professionally approved authorities. There was so much material to master that the specialist—considered a charlatan for much of the nineteenth century—was now the revered, often wealthy, consultant, whose domain as often as not was the hospital. No longer places only for the sick poor, hospitals were equipped with diagnostic facilities, surgical theaters, obstetric wards, and professional nurses, all organized and run according to the doctors' wishes. Doctors' wishes, moreover, carried far more weight now—reinforced, as they were, by science, by physical evidence, and by the demonstrable success of modern medicine in dealing with matters of health. Although some people (including some physicians) lamented the loss of the old-fashioned country doctor and the old-fashioned country practice,[3] and were dismayed by the white-coated, laboratory-oriented, impersonal antiseptic efficiency of the modern hospital and examining room, others held medicine and its recent accomplishments in awe. And although there were some who thought that public health officials, sanitary engineers, and better food ought to receive more credit, medical science and medical men generally received most of the accolades. Overseeing it all was the AMA—not without opposition or criticism, but the AMA's efforts had helped transform the rather motley collection of turn-of-the-century practitioners into a powerful, sovereign profession. Sectarian practices faded from the scene (though not completely). Medical knowledge was now far too esoteric, its practices far too complex, and its medicines far too potent for the average layperson to understand or implement in home care. Major illnesses were clearly treated more effectively by physicians, who "finally had medical practice pretty much to themselves."[4]

Pharmacy, too, had achieved some of its professional goals in these decades (notably in educating and licensing pharmacy graduates),[5] and the World's Fair highlighted the often- overlooked contributions druggists had made to medicine and to public health. But although pharmacists were respectable enough, they did not have the cachet of physicians, and the exigencies of the retail business often worked against professional ideals. Physicians found their professionalism enhanced by the contemporary advances in science; pharmacists, in fact, found theirs diminished. The fashion for factory-made and packaged drugs had only increased after the turn of the century, and it became exceeding rare for any druggist to dispense any prescription from scratch. Virtually all the medicinal items in an American drugstore after World War I came from large, industrial manufacturers, often bearing patents and certainly bearing trade names, the best of them more likely now to be American rather than German. For the American pharmaceutical industry had also come into its own in these years, taking advantage of wartime disruption of the German companies, focusing to some extent on the production of biologicals (with which they already had experience) rather than synthetics, and providing innovative products that could compete with even the best European drugs.[6] The industrial research laboratory was now well established in the United States and was already responsible for about half of new drug discoveries and for converting the other half from raw ideas into marketable, clinically useful items.[7] Few of these institutions, however, were represented at the Chicago pavilion, for the organizers had refused to accept exhibitors who made unsupported claims for their products and apparently did not want the displays to resemble trade show advertising.

Although much of the credit for medical progress could be associated with the pharmaceutical industry, the features of the industry that had troubled the medical world at the turn of the century had not changed significantly; if anything, the trade had become more sophisticated and troublesome. Advertisements masquerading as medical articles, free samples and other inducements, and extravagant and unsupported claims were not just to be found in the pages of *Cosmopolitan* or the *Daily News*. (Only since 1962, after the passage of the Kefauver-Harris Amendment to the Food, Drug, and Cosmetic Act of 1938, did the efficacy of drugs have to be demonstrated.) Medical journals were still in need of advertising revenues, and busy doctors who may have graduated from medical school some years earlier were still in need of succinct information on the latest products. They could most easily find it in the manufacturers' material. In 1946 this culminated in the *Physicians' Desk Reference*, which has remained the most popular guide to available drugs but is not an independent evaluation of pharmaceutical products. Rather, it is "a promotional device," and the information it contains is supplied by the drug companies.[8]

Nonetheless, over the course of the twentieth century, manufacturers have provided a host of medicines for which practitioners (and patients) are extremely appreciative. In the fifty years after the Chicago World's Fair, a veritable flood of important new drugs opened up a whole new era in medical practice: antibiotics, tranquilizers, steroids, antipsychotics, antihypertensives, contraceptives, beta-blockers. For all its faults, the pharmaceutical industry has been responsible for many of the products that allow the medical profession (with all *its* faults) to remain sovereign and powerful.[9] If we had to judge medicine's progress in the twentieth century only by the headache, however, we might reach a different conclusion.

There was no "eureka" moment in headache studies, no breakthrough drug or universal treatment, no discovery that unlocked the key to understanding this affliction. It remained puzzling, persistent, difficult to categorize, and frustrating to treat. Millions of Americans in the twentieth century continued to suffer debilitating headaches of one sort or another, and doctors still did not really know why. Only the "ordinary" headache was seemingly conquered, or at least was fought to a draw—by aspirin. This was no small accomplishment, certainly, and countless more millions of Americans were grateful for it. But aspirin was not a cure, it was only a palliative, and it afforded few insights into why headaches happened in the first place.[10]

Even more significantly, because of aspirin's success as a home remedy, physicians rather reluctantly began to abandon the position that every headache needed a proper diagnosis before treatment, although it was not until after World War II that they would admit publicly that "There is no valid reason why the lay individual should be forced to consult a physician and secure a prescription if he wants to obtain some aspirin for the temporary relief of an occasional headache."[11] But of course the lay individual had long ago made this determination for himself. By the early 1920s, in fact, it was apparent that over-the-counter analgesics had relegated most headaches to the status of minor inconveniences and that most doctors were happy enough to leave them there. There were, after all, far more serious medical challenges that they needed to address. But this meant that only persons with chronic and severe headaches visited their physicians. To some extent this had always been true, and headache cases had been among the most exasperating in any practice, but the headaches themselves had been taken seriously: the ailment was believed to be rooted in some mysterious but physically real cause. The new division of headaches into those for which aspirin worked and those for which it did not, however, helped create a different perspective, a new lens through which to view this aggravating complaint and, by extension, the complainer. Headache research and treatments as they developed after about 1920 are to a significant extent a reflection of this shift in attitude. Although the history of the headache since World War I is far more multifaceted, complex, and involved than we can do justice to here, we can paint its broad outlines with reasonable clarity.

Headache research after the Great War continued in much the same vein as before. Identifying and eliminating causes was still more important than treating the symptoms. Eyestrain, nasal and sinus problems, circulatory ailments, toxins, fatigue, preexisting diseases, and especially gastric misadventure were still the most common culprits, but as in the nineteenth century, the number of possible causes was long and unwieldy, and the clever but fairly Byzantine classification schemes some doctors proposed were not altogether helpful—although perhaps everyone could support in principle the categories suggested by a British doctor: headaches with pain one can forget, those with pain one cannot forget, and those with pain that makes one forget everything else.[12]

Nevertheless, in the period between the two world wars, some

dedicated neurologists as well as specialists in various other disciplines
continued to gather data, evaluate possible pain mechanisms, and explore
various treatment possibilities. One of the more important breakthroughs
in the 1920s was the serendipitous observation that preparations of ergot
(a fungus that grows on rye) were often useful in aborting migraine.[13] Ergo-
tamine tartrate quickly became standard migraine treatment, although it
was not until the 1930s that an American researcher explored the reasons
for its effectiveness. Harold Wolff, a neurologist at Cornell, determined
that migraine pain was the result of the dilation of the blood vessels of the
brain.[14] Ergot, a vasoconstrictor, interrupted this process. This vascular
theory of migraine was generally accepted for the next fifty or more years
and became the foundation for much subsequent research. Yet ergot, too,
was merely a symptomatic remedy. Why the blood vessels dilated was not
known. Indeed, Wolff postulated that the first stage of migraine (the sco-
toma or flashing lights that occur about twenty minutes before the pain
sets in) was due to the very vasoconstriction that seemed to cure the second stage. In the space of half an hour, two apparently contradictory phenomena occurred, without any obvious trigger for either of them.

The absence of identifiable physical causes in the vast majority of
headaches was a predicament for a medical profession whose success and
authority were now wedded to mechanistic principles, to quantifiable, tan-
gible, and visible evidence of illness. Yet 90 percent of headaches had no
x-rays, no blood tests, no laboratory findings to confirm their existence,
much less to suggest why they happened. Fortunately, because most headaches were "ordinary," the failure to understand their causes was of no
great moment: they disappeared soon enough, and even sooner upon taking aspirin.[15] But there remained that other large population whose pain
was so severe or so frequent that over-the-counter painkillers had no
effect. By the time these people had consulted a physician, they had often
tried every treatment available. In a small percentage of cases the problem
might turn out to be an injury, an infected tooth, a pinched nerve, or other
condition for which the doctor had a workable solution. Yet in most
instances of severe headache, medical science was still not able to determine the headache's ultimate cause, far less provide a specific remedy. As
a result, physicians could not often offer treatment that was any more
effective than what the patient could do at home—with the possible excep-

tion of narcotics. As custodians of the opiates, physicians did have the power to provide quick and effective relief in dire instances.

Although narcotics had never been thought appropriate in garden-variety headaches, in the nineteenth century their use in serious pain had been acceptable and humane. In the wake of the Harrison Narcotic Act, however, when addiction became a crime and prescribers therefore could become criminals, American physicians were concerned that they might be accused of dope trafficking if they were too free with their prescriptions. Because small amounts of narcotics were still available in over-the-counter nostrums (until 1970), headache victims tended to consult doctors only when they wanted larger doses, but now the physician might suspect the patient of "drug-seeking behavior" rather than genuine physical problems. Reluctance to prescribe narcotics thus became and has remained a feature of the American medical profession, even as pain control remains the one well-established, workable method of treating a bad headache.[16] And patients with bad headaches thus became the bane of many a doctor.

Among the various innovations that medical thought had produced around 1900, however, one in particular was poised to provide an altogether new perspective on headaches, a perspective that many in the medical profession eventually embraced as a potential solution to the headache dilemma—psychiatry. In the first decades of the twentieth century, this relatively new specialty was beginning to offer some attractive explanations for headaches and other ailments that seemed to have no physical causes. The mind had long been accepted in Western medicine as playing an important role in disease. Conscious emotions such as fear, worry, or anger were known to influence a person's health, but because emotions—that is, one's temperament—were themselves the products of the humors or the constitution, the mind–body connection retained a certain physicality. One's constitution, in a sense, created one's personality. Nervous people had weak or sensitive nervous systems, and were "neurotic" only because the word was related to "nerves." When, however, Sigmund Freud, Georg Groddeck, and other pioneers in the study of the mind introduced concepts such as the unconscious and the subconscious, repression, suppression, sublimation, conversion hysteria, and other psychic phenomena, new explanatory mechanisms became available: headaches could now be explained as psychogenic or psychosomatic disease. One's personality now created one's constitution. Psychic trauma, unresolved conflicts, repressed urges, and other emotional struggles that often originated in childhood displayed themselves as somatic afflictions, ulcers, palpitations, headaches. "Neurotic" now meant "associated with the mental states," and a headache that had no other discernable cause could be described as the "symbolic expression [of] sexual repression of childhood" or the "repression of hostile aggressive impulses."[17]

Although these theories of mind were complex, multifaceted, and competitive within the psychiatric community, the headache as a manifestation of neurosis in this new sense became fairly widely accepted by the 1930s.[18] A neurotic headache victim had a personality disorder. Perhaps he had "the 'soul' of a child, unwilling to endure the arbitrary limitations of his present life"; perhaps he had developed his neuroses out of selfishness.[19] Investigators suggested that headaches were the result of "hatred of beloved persons," with associated "mental castration" of the beloved's head, and other Oedipal images.[20] The long-standing connection between headaches and nasal problems could now be accounted for by the fact that "the nose is a sexual organ" that has "emotional states" and that "the interior structures of the nose reflect emotional pathology." Just as some people get sick because they subconsciously refuse to have a bowel movement, others get headaches because they subconsciously refuse to let their sinuses drain.[21] Even if sexual meanings were absent, psychogenic headaches at the very least were likely the "guilt-relieving self-absorption of projected feelings of hostility" toward a spouse, child, boss, or colleague.[22]

Migraine proved to be particularly suitable for psychiatric explanations. Harold Wolff, in addition to determining migraine's vascular features, also developed a "migraine personality" profile, which was very influential in subsequent migraine and other headache research. His 1937 study of twenty-five female and twenty-one male migraine sufferers found that many had been "delicate" as children, had been shy, obedient but stubborn, liked by their teachers, careful with their toys, tidy, and exceptionally attached to their mothers. As adults they were ambitious, meticulous, inflexible, and perfectionist. Two-thirds of the sample "harbored strong resentments" toward someone. Four-fifths of the women were dissatisfied with their sex lives. All the subjects were easily provoked, found their work frustrating, and could not relax easily. In all of them it was evident there was an "increase in stress produced by clearly definable life situations."[23] Later, he described the "pernicious way of life" of the typical migraineur as one of "resentment, tension, fatigue and exhaustion."[24] Migraine sufferers could not express their real feelings, so they turned them in on themselves and had a headache instead of an argument.

Furthermore, as other investigators noted, the preponderance of female migraine sufferers could now "probably be accounted for by the fact that in so many ways women are more sensitive than men and more inclined to be prostrated by discomforts. . . . When a man has an attack of migraine, he usually takes some headache powder and goes on with his work, while his sisters with the same disease and inheritance may have to go home to bed." This author hastened to add that this was "not intended as a disparagement of women or their fortitude; it is just a statement of facts as they are noted by physicians." But he also noted that "many a woman with migraine gets a bad attack simply from planning a bridge party or a tea or a dinner or a journey. Others are constantly worn out because they can't make up their minds quickly, and every shopping trip becomes an ordeal. . . . Obviously, no physician can hope to help these patients so long as they keep wearing themselves out in all these foolish ways." Clearly, "such women must do their best to reform and break a lot of bad psychic habits." A new job or marriage to a man "who would love her and make life easy for her" would probably cure her, too.[25] Her headache—although physically real—was all in her head, a classic psychosomatic affliction that women were more prone to because of the attributes of their sex. Is it any wonder women now felt they and their headaches were not being taken seriously?

Migraines were not confined to women, however, and men with the same personality traits who reached a point where they could not "cope with the accumulating tension and hostility resulting from the stress" in their lives likewise produced a vascular reaction and a headache. This response to the environment "serve[d] to remove the individual from the threat or the threat from the individual."[26] The demonstrated involvement of the blood vessels proved that the headache was not fictitious. Yet in some cases, as another author noted, the pain might indeed be "in the form of a delusion or hallucination," real to the patient but "false to everyone around him." Such patients were often "extremely self-centered,"

doing "anything to 'get their way' or sometimes to 'get attention.' An
example of this is that they will complain of a severe headache attack
merely to get the attention or the sympathy of their mate or their friends."
Unfortunately, "this type of personality is often found to be the type which
is incapable of loving anyone or anything very deeply but himself." Such
persons are also usually anxious and insecure, or worried and frustrated,
and have nothing "to think about but themselves." They need something
to complain about, and "it seems that headache is all too frequently chosen as the disturbance" to focus on. The problem is not quite all in the
mind, however. "Most of these patients, who are correctly diagnosed as
having psychogenic headaches, simply do not have a nervous system
which can cope with the ordinary demands of everyday life, and because of
this strain, there is a breakdown and the psychoneurosis presents itself.
This may occur at practically any stage in life from childhood on through
adulthood."[27] This author also stressed the need to eliminate all other
causes before settling on a psychogenic diagnosis and thought that many
psychogenic headaches were misdiagnosed. Other physicians, however,
thought that "headache of emotional origin [was] probably more common
than most of us realize," particularly recurrent types. Because the pain
might appear long after the trigger, causal connections were difficult to
determine. Even when a connection was made, it might be misconstrued.
Parties and other gatherings often precipitated a headache, for which the
victim blamed the noise, or smoke, or lights, but in fact it was the social
stress of the occasion.[28]

Psychological explanations were also invoked for other, lesser forms of
headache—even when the mechanism was determined to be physical, as
in the tension headache. Once again, Harold Wolff was responsible for
establishing the criteria, based in part on experiments conducted in the
1940s that produced pain in subjects whose head and neck muscles were
contracted. Because many emotional states produce clenching of the neck
and facial muscles, it was but a short step to connecting the vast majority
of otherwise-unexplained headaches to a psychological cause. The garden-
variety headache was now the tension headache. Even when the primary
cause was physical, if therapy (including analgesics) failed, the patient's
inability to cope and poor adjustment to life could then be blamed. In fact,

in some instances it was taken as diagnostic that if aspirin did not work, the patient was neurotic.[29]

Despite the growing popularity of psychological explanations, some practitioners were leery of the psychogenic headache, seeing it as "a smooth diagnosis with which to gloss over contemporaneous difficulties. In time, it ripples off the tongue so readily that it requires no cerebral process to guide its use. . . . [It] is admirably adapted to the needs of the hurried practitioner."[30] The associated treatment, however, was not. Psychotherapy, especially psychoanalysis, was meant to be a fairly prolonged affair in which all aspects of the patient's past, his dreams, his family relationships, marriage, work, and recreation were explored. In effect, the doctor had to alter the patient's personality.[31] At the very least, the sufferer had to be made aware of the underlying conflicts that were manifesting themselves as headaches. It was not an approach that promised a quick fix, and it demanded a great deal of the physician as well as of the patient, although sometimes a thorough case history was all that was necessary to produce relief. But many Americans did not welcome a psychological diagnosis, even when the migraine personality flattered them by being associated with high intelligence and creativity. (Freud himself, Darwin, and Caesar were all said to have had migraines.) "It must be remembered that the laity still look on neuroses as shameful and dishonest, and on organic illness as bearing no stigma."[32] "There are still millions of people to whom seeing a psychiatrist means that they 'must be crazy,' and millions more to whom the idea of treating a 'real pain' by just talking seems the most arrant nonsense."[33] Patients were convinced that the source of their throbbing temples was organic, but the psychogenic category nevertheless remained attractive to practitioners who were frankly stymied by the persistent difficulties in determining other kinds of causes. Unfortunately, whatever physicians actually thought of their headache patients and their pain, the patients themselves often felt that they were treated unsympathetically, dismissed as weak willed, immature, mentally unstable, or drug addicts.

This is not to say that investigators gave up research into physical diagnoses. In 1948 the indefatigable Harold Wolff published what quickly became the standard text in the field. *Headache and Other Head Pain* incorporated his earlier findings on migraine, as well as other work, much of it devoted to determining pain mechanisms and pain pathways, identifying the structures involved, and pursuing headaches that were clearly related to some physical cause: headaches of trauma, brain tumors, sinus infection, nerve degeneration, infections, and so on.[34] Wolff was of course not alone in his pursuits. By the late 1950s, in fact, the need to "bring together men practicing in the various fields of medicine so that they may express their ideas and beliefs about various forms of headache and head pain" resulted in the foundation of the American Association for the Study of the Headache (recently renamed the American Headache Society), whose journal *Headache* became the first periodical devoted to the subject. Despite the dedicated work of many individuals in the United States and elsewhere,[35] however, it would be difficult to point to any significant advances either in the fundamentals of headache pathology or in innovative or effective treatments until the late 1980s, when, among other things, investigations into the neurotransmitter serotonin led to the development of sumatriptan (Imitrex) as a migraine treatment, and the tricyclic antidepressants such as amitriptyline were found to be effective in tension-type headaches. Headache researchers themselves acknowledge these discoveries as auspicious, because they are predicated on findings in brain chemistry, genetics, and other basic sciences and show much promise. They also bring relief (in more than one sense) to headache sufferers for whom these data are proof of the essentially biological basis of their affliction. Simultaneously, in fact, psychogenic explanations have become rarer, and the long-standing psychological basis for the classic tension headache (which recent research had actually shown does not necessarily involve clenched muscles and therefore is now called the tension-type headache) has been called "a prejudiced and unproven allegation."[36] Psychiatry is still important in current practice, but rather than explore issues of repressed hostility or the sexual symbolism of noses, it tends to help patients cope with the invalidism and frustration that accompany their headaches, because, unfortunately, the new treatments have not been effective in all cases. For every success, there is someone else with an intractable migraine. Headache pathology is still largely terra incognita.

What is less uncertain, however, is the extent to which the American medical profession now controls the options available to this portion of the headache population. The 1951 Humphrey-Durham amendment finally eliminated public access to whole classes of drugs; in 1970, all remaining narcotics were removed from over-the-counter products. Although patients are free to consult naturopaths, chiropractors, acupuncturists, and other alternative practitioners, they must obtain the new headache remedies from a regular doctor by means of a prescription, and in an emergency, only a physician can authorize the Demerol or morphine that can alleviate the attack. A time-traveling doctor from an earlier era might be well pleased at this turn of events. At last physicians have a de facto monopoly over powerful yet dangerous drugs. Their knowledge protects ignorant laypersons from harming themselves.

But our visitor from the past might also be very concerned about the role the pharmaceutical industry plays in contemporary headache treatment, and might be forgiven for supposing that turn-of-the-century predictions of manufacturing druggists taking over medical practice and of commercial interests interfering with medical decisions had in fact come to pass. Although the intimate and often troubling association of doctors and the drug trade as it developed in the twentieth century has only been explored in part, it takes its direction from elements we have already encountered. For one thing, patents are now standard operating procedure with all new drugs and make the headache medicines extremely expensive, beyond the reach of many patients. For another, advertising remains the principal method of informing the medical profession about the product. Moreover, some prescription-only drugs have recently been advertised to the laity, acquainting them with their brand names and sometimes their applications—more reason for our time traveler to wonder who's in charge.

Certainly the part of the population that suffers from ordinary headaches has more cause to be grateful to the drug manufacturers than to the medical profession, if we accept that quick relief from headache pain is desirable (although it was various Food and Drug legislation that compelled the industry to pay more attention to safety issues). At any rate, acetanilid powders remained on the market, and phenacetin was still widely available until the late 1970s, usually in combination with aspirin and caffeine (the APC formulation), when the FDA proscribed the use of these aniline-based drugs in the United States. In the interim, however, various new aspirin combinations (notably Excedrin and Bufferin) had become nationally known brands and were challenging Bayer and Anacin. In the 1950s, acetaminophen came to America as Tylenol, with analgesic properties equivalent to those of aspirin but with no gastric side effects. It did not become popular until the 1970s, however, when a new advertising campaign told consumers that "you can't buy a more potent pain reliever without a prescription."[37] At about the same time, a prescription pain reliever from the class of drugs known as nonsteroidal anti-inflammatories (NSAIDs) was reaching the end of its patent, and its makers persuaded the FDA to approve it for over-the-counter use. Thus in 1984 several companies began marketing ibuprofen under various trade names: Motrin and Advil became the best known. These were followed by other NSAIDs, and although all have some potential for gastric irritation and are not harmless if abused, they have found much favor among people needing moderate pain relief. They are agreeably priced and widely available, with sales now averaging around two billion dollars a year. These drugs do not, of course, cure a headache, but they work well enough in many cases. In some important sense they connect present-day Americans to a long tradition of self-diagnosis and self-treatment.

Clearly, the headache is still a challenge on all levels. Pain control, although it is probably what patients desire most and would be happiest with, is still not the primary goal of medical researchers, who continue to look for the underlying pathology in order that therapies be based on rational principles. Recent innovations in the use of antidepressants have produced optimism in both the research and patient communities, but these therapies are not panaceas. For the millions of Americans for whom over-the-counter or even prescription drugs are not effective (the indiscriminate use of painkillers has in fact led to the "rebound headache"), self-help groups, chat lines, information exchanges, and newsletters can provide coping strategies. Indeed, these groups also try to educate those physicians and health care personnel who still think a headache is not "a legitimate biological disease" and who seem to populate many emergency rooms and family practices, if patients' stories on the Internet are representative of prevailing attitudes.[38] New technologies notwithstanding, the diagnosis of headache requires that the physician believe what the patient is saying. Apparently there is still a credibility gap. And apparently there is also a sympathy gap. Successful treatment of headache requires that practitioners (and friends and family members) appreciate that pain itself can be as devastating as any disease.

It is highly unlikely that the headache will ever go the way of smallpox or even neurasthenia and become a quaint reminder of times past, of an ignorant and helpless era in medical history. But it is very likely that whatever solutions are found, they will be the result of the cooperation and commiseration of sufferers, physicians, and industry alike, and that sooner or later, we will find some of them for sale in our corner drugstore.

NOTES

INTRODUCTION

1. One of Jefferson's most informative references was in a letter he wrote in June 1790 to his daughter Martha about a recent headache: it had been "very violent for a few days" but had soon subsided and could "hardly be called a pain now, but only a disagreeable sensation of the head every morning." Thomas Jefferson, *The Family Letters of Thomas Jefferson*, ed. E. M. Botts and J. A. Bear (Columbia: University of Missouri Press, 1966), 58.

2. It is in fact a late twentieth-century biographer who brings up a possible psychological explanation for these headaches, noting that they occurred at stressful periods of Jefferson's life. Fawn Brodie, *Thomas Jefferson: An Intimate History* (New York: Norton, 1974), 43.

3. Robert Ferrell, ed., *The Eisenhower Diaries* (New York: Norton, 1981), 43, 215–216.

4. *American Heritage Dictionary of the English Language*, 3rd ed. (Boston: Houghton-Mifflin, 1992), 831.

5. John Steinbeck, *The Wayward Bus* (New York: Viking Press, 1947). Mrs. Pritchard and her headache can be found in chapter 13.

CHAPTER 1   THE HEADACHE AND ITS TREATMENT IN THE NINETEENTH CENTURY

1. Ulysses S. Grant, *Personal Memoirs of U. S. Grant* (New York: Charles L. Webster, 1885–1886), 2:483–485; Ulysses S. Grant, *Memoirs and Selected Letters* (New York: Library of America, 1990), 390, 943, 952, 971; Bruce Catton, *Grant Takes Command* (Boston: Little, Brown, 1969), 459–460.

2. Mary Chesnut, *Mary Chesnut's Civil War*, ed. C. V. Woodward (New Haven: Yale University Press, 1981). Her 4 July headache is referred to on p. 832; her angelic neighbor on p. 344; angina and other ailments, passim. Alcohol was also recognized as having painkilling properties, but its effectiveness was limited and seems to have been achieved mostly by making the patient drunk. Moreover, its use was far more likely to result in a headache than cure one.

3. Feeling particularly cheerful one day in 1889, she asked if her nurse might not like to trade places with her. "Inside of you, Miss," replied the other woman,

"when you have just had a sick head-ache for five days!" James's own diary apparently does not record this headache. Leon Edel, ed., *The Diary of Alice James* (New York: Dodd, Mead, 1964), 48

4. Henry James, *Selected Letters*, ed. Leon Edel (Cambridge: Harvard University Press, 1987), 45. He refers to an "intestinal drama" of late 1869 (62).

5. Louisa May Alcott, *Selected Letters of Louisa May Alcott*, ed. Joel Myerson and Daniel Shealy (Boston: Little, Brown, 1987), 305–306.

6. Henry James, *The American* (1879; reprint, London: John Lehmann, 1949), 23.

7. Lansford P. Yandell, "On the Bromide of Potassium in Headache and Epilepsy," *American Practitioner* 1 (1870): 84.

8. Lillian Schlissel, *Women's Diaries of the Westward Journey* (New York: Schocken Books, 1982), 206.

9. Pain is as much a cultural phenomenon as a physical one, and how pain affects individuals is often discussed in psychological, philosophical, or sociological rather than strictly biological terms. The religious meaning of pain is examined by C. S. Lewis, *The Problem of Pain* (London: Geoffrey Bles, 1940), and its transformation to a secular phenomenon by Donald Caton, "The Secularization of Pain," *Anesthesiology* 62 (1985): 493–501. For an exploration of the politics of suffering and the theme that the meanings of pain are socially constructed, see David B. Morris, *The Culture of Pain* (Berkeley: University of California Press, 1991); and Elaine Scarry, *The Body in Pain: The Making and Unmaking of the World* (New York: Oxford University Press, 1985). See also Joseph Kotarba, *Chronic Pain: Its Social Dimensions* (Beverly Hills, Calif.: Sage Publications, 1983), which summarizes various sociological models. The role of physicians as mediators of suffering is examined by Eric Cassell, *The Nature of Suffering and the Goals of Medicine* (New York: Oxford University Press, 1991). For a historical perspective, see James Turner, *Reckoning with the Beast: Animals, Pain and Humanity in the Victorian Mind* (Baltimore: Johns Hopkins University Press, 1980). See also Elizabeth B. Clark, " 'The Sacred Rights of the Weak': Pain, Sympathy and the Culture of Individual Rights in Antebellum America," *Journal of American History* 82 (1985): 463–483. Martin Pernick, *A Calculus of Suffering: Pain, Professionalism, and Anesthesia in Nineteenth-Century America* (New York: Columbia University Press, 1985), examines medical attitudes to pain, but Pernick is primarily concerned with the role surgical anesthesia played in shaping the American medical profession, as physicians found themselves able to relieve certain profound kinds of suffering.

10. Collections of folk remedies can be found in Wayland D. Hand, *Magical Medicine* (Berkeley: University of California Press, 1980); and William George Black, *Folk-Medicine; A Chapter in the History of Culture* (1883; reprint, Nendeln, Liechtenstein: Kraus Reprints, 1967).

11. Mrs. E. F. Haskell, *Civil War Cooking*, ed. R. L. Shep (Mendocino, Calif.: R. L. Shep, 1992), 378; this volume is a facsimile of *The Housekeeper's Encyclopedia*, published in 1861.

12. William Glasgow, "On Certain Measures for the Relief of Congestive Headaches," *New York Medical Journal* 46 (1887): 260–262.

13. In the litany of illnesses suffered by slaves and discussed by Julius Lester, *To Be a Slave* (New York: Scholastic Press, 1968), headache is not mentioned.

14. "Remarkable Case of a Young Gardener," *Gentleman's Magazine* 41 (1771): 152.

15. Thomas Jefferson, *The Family Letters of Thomas Jefferson*, ed. Edwin M. Botts and James A. Bear (Columbia: University of Missouri Press, 1966), 58.

16. William H. Day, *Headaches; Their Nature, Causes, and Treatment*, 3rd ed. (Philadelphia: Lindsay and Blakiston, 1880), 22.

17. See John S. Haller, Jr., *American Medicine in Transition, 1840–1910* (Urbana: University of Illinois Press, 1981). Chap. 1 offers an excellent summary of medical ideas at the beginning of the nineteenth century.

18. See, for example, Gert Brieger, "Therapeutic Conflicts and the American Medical Profession in the 1860s," *Bulletin of the History of Medicine* 41 (1967): 215–222. Medical education is discussed further in chap. 3.

19. James Harley Warner, *The Therapeutic Perspective: Medical Practice, Knowledge, and Identity in America, 1820–1885* (Cambridge: Harvard University Press, 1986), 85. Warner's excellent study clearly points out the diversity of opinions and points of view among practitioners and their ambivalence about the impact of experimental science on their profession. For a nineteenth-century view, see J. Russell Reynolds, ed., *A System of Medicine*, 3rd ed. (London: Macmillan, 1876), 1:1.

20. A very informative discussion of these matters can be found in Charles E. Rosenberg, " 'Therapeutic Revolution': Medicine, Meaning, and Social Change in Nineteenth Century America," in Morris J. Vogel and Charles E. Rosenberg, eds., *The Therapeutic Revolution: Essays in the Social History of American Medicine* (Philadelphia: University of Pennsylvania Press, 1979).

21. William Cullen, *The Works of William Cullen, M.D.*, ed. J. Thomson, 2 vols. (Edinburgh: William Blackwood, 1827), 2:545.

22. Jean-Baptiste Burserius, *The Institutions of the Practice of Medicine*, trans. from the Latin by William Cullen Brown (Edinburgh: Cadell, 1800–1803), 4:1–45.

23. Ralph W. Leftwich, *An Index of Symptoms as a Clue to Diagnosis*, 2nd ed. (London: Smither, Elder, 1901), 21–23. Other contributions included classification systems based on the time the headache occurred (when awakening at night, or between midnight and morning, or between midnight and ten o'clock in the morning), each with a different remedy (left or right side was also important). John C. King, *Headaches and Their Concomitant Symptoms* (Chicago: W. A. Chatterton, 1879).

24. Jan R. McTavish, "The Headache in American Medical Practice in the Nineteenth Century: A Historical Overview," *Headache* 39 (1999): 287–298.

25. Yandell, "On the Bromide of Potassium," 83.

26. The problem of defining historical concepts of pain is a thorny one, as was

discussed in n. 9, but whether the pain was caused by injuries, disease, or God, doctors do not seem to have viewed it as "imagined."

27. Silas W. Mitchell, "Headaches from Heat-Stroke, from Fevers, after Meningitis, from Over Use of the Brain, from Eye Strain," *Medical and Surgical Reporter* 31 (1874): 67–70, 81–84; reprinted in *Headache* 3 (1963–1964): 70–76.

28. Day, *Headaches*, 22.

29. George B. Groff, "Headaches, and the Remedies Proposed," *Therapeutic Gazette* 5 (1881): 67.

30. See Daniel W. Cathell, *Book on the Physician Himself and Things That Concern His Reputation and Success*, 10th ed. (Philadelphia: F. A. Davis, 1898), 276. A proposal in California to allow prescriptions in English if the patient wanted it was called "ridiculous." "Writing Prescriptions in English," *Medical Record* 17 (1880): 344.

31. George Wood, "General Therapeutics," in *A Treatise on the Practice of Medicine*, 3rd ed., 2 vols. (Philadelphia: Lippincott, Grambo, 1852), 1:206ff.

32. It was nevertheless one of the most powerful therapeutic options doctors possessed. Its uses are summarized by James Wardrop, *On the Curative Effects of the Abstraction of Blood, with Rules for Employing both Local and General Blood-Letting in the Treatment of Diseases* (Philadelphia: A. Waldie, 1837).

33. Wood, "General Therapeutics," 1, 206ff.

34. See Alfred Stillé, *Therapeutics and Materia Medica*, rev. 3rd ed., 2 vols. (Philadelphia: Henry C. Lea, 1868), 1:94–98. In addition, American disease was different from European simply because of the difference in the locale. D. G. Brinton, "Therapeutics as a Local Art," *Medical and Surgical Reporter* 35 (1876): 386–387.

35. The concept is summarized by Alex Berman, "The Heroic Approach in Nineteenth-Century Therapeutics," *Bulletin of the American Society of Hospital Pharmacists* 11 (1954): 320–327.

36. Maurice Clarke, "Therapeutic Nihilism," *Boston Medical and Surgical Journal* 119 (1888): 199–201.

37. Phyllis Allen, "Etiological Theory in America Prior to the Civil War," *Journal of the History of Medicine and Allied Sciences* 2 (1947): 489–520.

38. See Warner, *Therapeutic Perspective*, 7.

39. Edward John Waring, *A Manual of Practical Therapeutics*, 2nd ed. (London: Churchill, 1865), 9. See also Otto Wall, *The Prescription: Therapeutically, Pharmaceutically, Grammatically and Historically Considered* (St. Louis: C. V. Mosby, 1917); John S. Haller, "With a Spoonful of Sugar: The Art of Prescription Writing in the Nineteenth and Early Twentieth Century," *Pharmacy in History* 26 (1984): 171–178.

40. James Mease, "On the Sick Headache," *Philadelphia Journal of Medical and Physical Sciences* 5 (1822): 1–23.

41. "Headache: A Few Suggestions," *American Journal of Clinical Medicine* 24 (1917): 90–91.

42. J. Leonard Corning, *A Treatise on Headache and Neuralgia* (New York: E. B. Treat, 1888), 34.

43. Various cures are summarized in McTavish, "Headache in American Medical Practice."

44. J. S. Jewell, "The Nature and Treatment of Headaches," *Journal of Nervous and Mental Diseases* 8 (1881): 64–79, 307–316. Jewell considered that a complete migraine cure would take at least "six months to two years of faithful attention to all reasonable details of treatment." He did, however, recommend opiates for particularly bad headaches.

45. T. S. Robertson, "Antipyrine in Migraine, Pyrexia, Etc.," *Medical Record* 31 (1887): 517–518.

46. T. Curtis Smith, "A Talk about Sick Headache," *Detroit Lancet* 8 (1884–1885): 339–342. Smith thought the gastric symptoms were ultimately dependent on the neurotic temperament of the patient but that good habits would prevent their occurrence.

47. Mease, "On the Sick Headache."

48. J. M. Scudder, "A Brief History of Eclectic Medicine," *Eclectic Medical Journal* 39 (1879): 297–308; Alex Berman, "A Striving for Scientific Respectability: Some American Botanics and the Nineteenth Century Plant Materia Medica," *Bulletin of the History of Medicine* 30 (1956): 7–31; John S. Haller, *Medical Protestants: The Eclectics in American Medicine, 1825–1939* (Carbondale: Southern Illinois University Press, 1994); John S. Haller, *The People's Doctor: Samuel Thomson and the American Botanical Movement, 1790–1860* (Carbondale: Southern Illinois University Press, 2000); Norman Gevitz, ed., *Other Healers: Unorthodox Medicine in America* (Baltimore: Johns Hopkins University Press, 1988).

49. W. S. Searle, "Headaches: From the Standpoint of a Subjective Symptom," *American Observer* 8 (1871): 33–38.

50. The entry for headache is about three and a half pages long (one of the longest): John H. Clarke, *The Prescriber: A Dictionary of the New Therapeutics*, 3rd ed. (London: Keene and Ashwell, 1889), 107–111. Similarly, a homeopathic treatment book of 1877 devoted 80 out of 1,500 pages to headache alone, more than to any other condition. See David Armstrong and Elizabeth Metzger-Armstrong, *The Great American Medicine Show* (New York: Prentice Hall, 1991), 33.

51. Headache "treatment has involved most of the drugs in the Pharmacopoeia and many additional measures"; Joseph Collins, "A Contribution to the Study of Headaches, with Particular Reference to their Etiology and Treatment," *Medical Record* 41 (1892): 370.

52. The lack of effective nonnarcotic analgesics meant that "the whole creation still groans and travails in pain"; H. W. Buxton, "The Philosophy of Pain," *Massachusetts Eclectic Medical Journal* 2 (1882): 103.

CHAPTER 2   DRUG SUPPLY IN NINETEENTH-CENTURY AMERICA

1.   J. E. Stewart, "Catarrh, Bronchitis, etc. . . . Popular Remedies," *Northern Lancet* 2 (1852): 23.

2.   Still the best comprehensive history of things pharmaceutical, including the drug trade, is Glenn Sonnedecker, ed., *Kremers and Urdang's History of Pharmacy*, 4th ed. (Philadelphia: Lippincott, 1976). See especially part 3, "Pharmacy in the United States." See also Jonathan Liebenau, *Medical Science and Medical Industry: The Formation of the American Pharmaceutical Industry* (Baltimore: Johns Hopkins University Press, 1987), chap. 2. Useful despite its lack of scholarly apparatus is Tom Mahoney, *The Merchants of Life: An Account of the American Pharmaceutical Industry* (New York: Harper and Brothers, 1959). Also see Gregory Higby and Elaine Stroud, eds., *The Inside Story of Medicines: A Symposium* (Madison, Wis.: American Institute for the History of Pharmacy, 1997).

3.   See John Ayrton Paris, *Pharmacologia*, 4th American ed., from the 7th British ed. (New York: W. E. Dean, 1831), 171.

4.   An excellent study of nineteenth-century pharmacy, including material on drug supply, can be found in Lee Anderson, *Iowa Pharmacy, 1880–1905: An Experiment in Professionalism* (Iowa City: University of Iowa Press, 1989). The first chapter provides a good introduction and overview.

5.   See Guenter B. Risse, Ronald L. Numbers, and Judith W. Leavitt, eds., *Medicine without Doctors: Home Health Care in American History* (New York: Science History Publications, 1977).

6.   One of the earliest federal regulations applied to drugs was the 1848 Drug Importation Act, which empowered U.S. customs officials to prevent adulterated foreign drugs from entering the country. It did not, however, provide any means to guarantee the purity of homegrown items. See Sonnedecker, *History of Pharmacy*, 219.

7.   *Fayette Watch Tower*, 4 January 1856.

8.   This is not to say that physicians were not active on their own behalf, and some doctors even encouraged domestic practice by writing books that provided practical advice for home care, yet all the while they emphasized that serious illness and injury should be treated by a regular practitioner. These medical guides, in fact, did a thriving business and helped reshape "the accepted boundaries of lay and professional medical responsibilities"; Lamar Riley Murphy, *Enter the Physician: The Transformation of Domestic Medicine, 1760–1860* (Tuscaloosa: University of Alabama Press, 1991), xv. Nevertheless, too much knowledge in the hands of the laity might create a population confident in its ability to heal itself. "Such notions clashed with the medical elite"; Michael A. Flannery, "Trouble in Paradise: A Brief Review of Therapeutic Contention in America, 1790–1864," *Pharmacy in History* 41 (1999): 153–163. For an overview of the American profession in this era, see Paul Starr, *The Social Transformation of American Medicine: The Rise of a Sovereign Profession and the Making of a Vast Industry* (New York: Basic Books, 1982), book 1.

9.   *Carpenter's Annual Medical Advertiser*, 1835.

10. Such ads appear, for example, in the *Jefferson Journal*, 1858, published in Jefferson County, Mississippi.

11. For discussions of the historical importance of homeopathy, see Robert Jütte, Guenter B. Risse, and John Woodward, eds., *Culture, Knowledge, and Healing: Historical Perspectives of Homeopathic Medicine in Europe and North America* (Sheffield, U.K.: European Association for the History of Medicine and Health Publications, 1998).

12. Tilden and Company of New York state and the W. S. Merrell and H. M. Merrell companies of Cincinnati were three of the most important. John S. Haller, *Medical Protestants: The Eclectics in American Medicine, 1825–1939* (Carbondale and Edwardsville: Southern Illinois University Press, 1994), 171.

13. See Murphy, *Enter the Physician*, esp. chap. 1; Norman Gevitz, "Domestic Medical Guides and the Drug Trade in Nineteenth Century America," *Pharmacy in History* 32 (1990): 51–56; Norman Gevitz, ed., *Other Healers: Unorthodox Medicine in America* (Baltimore: Johns Hopkins University Press, 1988); Charles Rosenberg, "Medical Text and Social Context: Explaining William Buchan's *Domestic Medicine*," *Bulletin of the History of Medicine* 57 (1983): 22–42.

14. *Boston Guide to Health and Journal of Arts and Sciences* 1 (1843).

15. *Botanic Investigator* 1 (1835): 16.

16. Benjamin Colby, *A Guide to Health* (Milford, N.H.: John Burns, 1846), 116. Colby said of opium: "It is the most common article used by those who wish to shuffle off this mortal coil" (28).

17. As a modern homeopathic text points out, "common sense dictates that pain has a value; it is a warning that there is something wrong. If our senses are dulled to the point that we cannot perceive pain, we may suffer serious consequences." Michael Weiner and Kathleen Goss, *The Complete Book of Homeopathy* (Garden City Park, N.Y.: Avery Publishing, 1989), 6.

18. For discussions on the meaning of pain, see n. 9 in chap. 1 of this volume.

19. Donald Caton, "The Secularization of Pain," *Anesthesiology* 63 (1985): 493–501.

20. Martin Pernick, *A Calculus of Suffering: Pain, Professionalism, and Anesthesia in Nineteenth-Century America* (New York: Columbia University Press, 1985), 72. Pernick calls the Painkiller "an entirely new concept in patent drugs." As we saw in the first chapter, professional medicine likewise found the idea novel, the word *analgesia* having usually meant "lethargy" up to this point.

21. However, Stewart Holbrook, *The Golden Age of Quackery* (New York: Macmillan, 1959), says it took forty years for Perry Davis's concoction to become famous (154).

22. Some early patent medicines were indeed granted patents, but lacking effective means to enforce the monopoly, they were immediately and universally imitated. Entrepreneurs therefore quickly discovered that it was more profitable

not to reveal their recipes (creating nostrums, i.e., "our" secret) and thereby establish the mystique of secret ingredients as an incentive to buy the product. The term *patent medicine*, however, remained attached to this class of goods from that day to this.

23. James Harvey Young, *The Toadstool Millionaires: A Social History of Patent Medi-cines in America before Federal Legislation* (Princeton: Princeton University Press, 1961), 110. A. Emil Hiss, *Thesaurus of Proprietary Preparations and Pharmaceutical Specialities* (Chicago: G. P. Engelhard, 1899), 9.

24. "Government Statistics Concerning Manufacturing Druggists," *Druggists Circu-lar* 51 (1907): 154–155.

25. Prospectus from the inaugural issue of *Guardian of Health* (Baltimore) 1 (1841): 1.

26. In addition to Young, *Toadstool Millionaires*, see also James Harvey Young, *The Medical Messiahs: A Social History of Health Quackery in Twentieth-Century America* (Princeton: Princeton University Press, 1967); James Harvey Young, *American Self-Dosage Medicines: An Historical Perspective* (Lawrence, Kan.: Coronado Press, 1974).

27. See, for example, the sympathetic portrait of Lydia Pinkham, in Sarah Stage, *Female Complaints: Lydia Pinkham and the Business of Women's Medicine* (New York: W. W. Norton, 1979). Also see Sarah Stage, "The Woman behind the Trademark," in *Women and Health in America: Historical Readings*, ed. Judith W. Leavitt (Madi-son: University of Wisconsin Press, 1984).

28. Frank Presbrey, *The History and Development of Advertising* (1929; reprint, New York: Greenwood Press, 1968), 289ff.; Pamela Walker Laird, "The Business of Progress: The Transformation of American Advertising, 1870–1920," 2 vols., Ph.D. dissertation, Boston University, 1992, 1:23ff.; Ralph M. Hower, *The History of an Advertising Agency: N. W. Ayer and Son at Work, 1869–1949*, rev. ed. (Cam-bridge: Harvard University Press, 1949), 44–46, 91–93. Hower discusses Ayer's increasingly negative view of the ethics of working with nostrum makers, despite the income it brought the agency. When the company finally dropped these clients in 1901, their patent medicine advertising revenue declined from $216,000 to $66,000 in one year. See also T. J. Jackson Lears, "From Salvation to Self-Realization: Advertising and the Therapeutic Roots of the Consumer Cul-ture, 1880–1930," in *The Culture of Consumption: Critical Essays in American His-tory, 1880–1980*, ed. Richard W. Fox and T. J. Jackson Lears (New York: Pantheon Books, 1983). Lears's interesting study of therapeutic imagery in turn-of-the-century advertising, however, does not examine what impact nostrum adver-tisements themselves might have had on this development. For examples of the splendor of nostrum advertising, see the fine collection of ads, trade cards, and other marketing paraphernalia in A. Walker Bingham, *The Snake Oil Syndrome: Patent Medicine Advertising* (Hanover, Mass.: Christopher Publishing House, 1994).

29. Laird, "Business of Progress," 1:30–32.

30. Young, *Toadstool Millionaires*, 190ff.

31. David Potter, *People of Plenty: Economic Abundance and the American Character* (Chicago: University of Chicago Press, 1954), 168ff. Potter notes that patent medicines used these devices long before any other products did.

32. Helen McKearin, *Bottles, Flasks and Dr. Dyott* (New York: Crown Publishers, 1970). Dyott was a Philadelphia entrepreneur who McKearin says was a marketer, not a mountebank.

33. Young, *Toadstool Millionaires*, 176ff. Not everyone was impressed: "Why a mixture of molasses, high wine, iron filings and cheap spices can claim absolute proprietorship to a common name simply because of the fact that the picture of a melancholy Indian adorns one side of the package and a mangy looking catamount or a moth-eaten squirrel the other, we know not"; "Trade-Marks," *Druggists Circular* 33 (1889): 60.

34. For a general history of the PAA, see Herbert Harding, "The History of Organization among Manufacturers and Wholesale Dealers in Proprietary Articles," *American Druggist* 36 (1900): 190–193; Young, *Toadstool Millionaires*, 107–108. The original name of the group was the Proprietary Medicine Manufacturers and Dealers Association. In 1990 it became the Nonprescription Drug Manufacturers Association (NDMA), and in 1999, the Consumer Health-Care Products Association (CHPA), located in Washington, D.C.

35. On the revenue from advertising, see Gerald J. Baldasty, *The Commercialization of News in the Nineteenth Century* (Madison: University of Wisconsin Press, 1992), 109–110. Also see Thomas Harrison Baker, *The Memphis Commercial Appeal: The History of a Southern Newspaper* (Baton Rouge: Louisiana University Press, 1971), 47; Young, *Toadstool Millionaires*, 82ff., 119ff.

36. Albert Prescott, "Should Proprietary Medicines Be Required to Give an Account of Contents?" *JAMA* 5 (1885): 132. See also James Harvey Young, "Federal Drug and Narcotic Legislation," *Pharmacy in History* 37 (1995): 59–67.

37. Minute Book, Proprietary Medicine Manufacturers and Dealers Association, December 1885, 140, CHPA, Washington, D.C.

38. The newspaper itself, however, may not have been quite as free in this matter as its readers. Like many papers, the *Globe* had a contract with the PAA that canceled patent medicine advertising if laws hostile to manufacturers were passed— the so-called red clause. It is not entirely clear, however, whether this clause was in effect in 1885. Louis M. Lyons, *Newspaper Story: One Hundred Years of the "Boston Globe"* (Cambridge: Harvard University Press, 1971), 158–159.

39. "Annual Meeting," PAA Minute Book, 25 September 1884, 115, CHPA, Washington, D.C.

40. The advertising material is available on microfilm: "Radway's Ready Relief," Canadian Institute for Historical Microreproductions (CIHM) 45896; "Paine's Celery Compound—Our Album," CIHM 32334; "Hamlin's Wizard Oil," CIHM 50670; "Griffith's Ready Reference and Etiquette Book," CIHM 41390.

41. J. Worth Estes, "The Pharmacology of Nineteenth-Century Patent Medicines," *Pharmacy in History* 30 (1988): 3–18.

42. Barbara Welch, "Being-in-Body: A Reflection upon American Self-Medication Drug Advertising," Ph.D. dissertation, University of Iowa, 1984, 89.

43. Pernick, *Calculus of Suffering*, 129.

44. David Musto, *The American Disease: Origins of Narcotic Control* (New Haven: Yale University Press, 1973), 3.

45. One analysis of Pinkham's Vegetable Compound gave the recipe as sixteen ounces of alcohol added to five pints of the base liquid, which was a concoction of various botanical ingredients (Hiss, *Thesaurus*, 222).

46. These figures were derived from my own unscientific count of the remedies in Hiss's *Thesaurus*. Of course, it may be that Hiss's catalog contains only the "respectable" proprietaries whose manufacturers by the turn of the century were more aware of the problems of narcotics addiction. At any given moment there appear to have been dozens of "fly-by-night" operations in the nostrum business, unconcerned with anything but turning a profit. Unregulated, they could concoct remedies with any amount of narcotics they wished.

47. W. F. McNutt, "Mrs. Winslow's Soothing Syrup—A Poison," *American Journal of Pharmacy* 44 (1872): 221–224; J. H. Salls, "The Proportion of Morphia in Winslow's Soothing Syrup," *American Journal of Pharmacy* 47 (1875): 482–483.

48. "Pain-Killers," *Cincinnati Lancet-Clinic* 7 (1881): 367, regarding an article by A. B. Prescott in *Physician and Surgeon*.

49. In 1889, however, the *Druggists Circular* published three possible formulas for the nostrum in response to a reader's request; only one recipe contained opium. "Perry Davis' Pain-Killer," *Druggists Circular* 33 (1889): 181.

50. "Nostrums Containing Habit Forming Drugs," *JAMA* 52 (1909): 1774.

51. R. F. Fairthorne, "Some Facts Concerning the Morphia and Opium Trade in the United States," *American Journal of Pharmacy* 52 (1880): 614–617.

52. David T. Courtwright, *Dark Paradise: Opiate Addiction in America before 1940* (Cambridge: Harvard University Press, 1982), 20. See also H. H. Kane, *Drugs That Enslave: The Opium, Morphine, Chloral and Hashisch Habits* (Philadelphia: Presley Blakiston, 1881).

53. George T. Welch, "Therapeutical Superstitions," *Medical Record* 44 (1893): 33–38.

54. George M. Beard, *American Nervousness: Its Causes and Consequences* (New York: Putnam's Sons, 1881); Benjamin Ward Richardson, *Diseases of Modern Life* (New York: D. Appleton, 1889). Richardson pointed out the problems stemming from a sedentary life, the use of tobacco, and overindulgence in food, drink, and the passions.

55. Courtwright, *Dark Paradise*, 36, and esp. 42–55, where he describes how and why the medical profession contributed to the problem. See also H. Wayne Morgan, *Yesterday's Addicts: American Society and Drug Abuse, 1865–1920* (Nor-

man: University of Oklahoma Press, 1974). A classic portrait of the respectable female addict is the character of the mother in Eugene O'Neill's *Long Day's Journey into Night*, a loosely autobiographical play, set in 1912. Addicts could also have gotten their start from any number of "legitimate" medications (paregoric, laudanum, Dover's powders), purchased with or without prescription from any drugstore or through the mail. Paradoxically, then, the very medical profession that was reluctant to treat pain such as a headache symptomatically was contributing to addiction to the most powerful painkillers in existence.

56. Easy access to narcotics had other hazards as well. The *New York Times* reported a "Melancholy Suicide with Laudanum" purchased at a neighborhood drugstore (29 September 1851, 2).

CHAPTER 3   DOCTORS AND THE DRUG TRADE

1. Arthur E. Hertzler, *The Horse and Buggy Doctor* (New York: Harper and Brothers, 1938), 34–37.

2. David L. Cowen, "Materia Medica and Pharmacology," in *The Education of American Physicians*, ed. Ronald Numbers (Berkeley: University of California Press, 1980), 100–105.

3. George Fox, *Reminiscences* (New York: Medical Life Press, 1926), 64.

4. Jacalyn Duffin's analysis of Langstaff's records indicate that although his therapeutic preferences changed to some extent over the thirty to forty years of his practice, he employed a fairly limited number of conventional therapies; opium, calomel, tartar emetic, and bloodletting predominated, although he often adjusted the prescription on a daily basis. (Unfortunately, he did not always tell us what he prescribed for the headaches.) Jacalyn Duffin, *Langstaff: A Nineteenth-Century Medical Life* (Toronto: University of Toronto Press, 1993). Daily prescribing seems to have been as common as the daily visit to the sick, according to other sources. David L. Cowen, Louis King, and Nicholas Lord, "Drug Use in the Nineteenth Century: A Computer Analysis," typescript, 1983, file C39q, Kremers Reference Files, University of Wisconsin, Madison.

5. Of twenty-one ethical companies established in the nineteenth century, only six existed before the Civil War. Dennis B. Worthen, "The Pharmaceutical Industry, 1852–1902," *Journal of the American Pharmaceutical Association* 40 (2000): 589–591.

6. Because most firms in the nineteenth century engaged in practices that even at the time raised eyebrows, their company histories are useful but usually not very self-critical. Typical "front-office" histories are Herman Kogan, *The Long White Line* (New York: Random House, 1963), on the Abbott company; and Leonard Engel, *Medicine Makers of Kalamazoo* (New York: McGraw-Hill, 1961) on Upjohn. See also John F. Marion, *The Fine Old House* (privately published, 1980), an anniversary history of Smith, Kline and French. Parke-Davis was favorably

reviewed by Frank O. Taylor, "Parke, Davis and Company," *Journal of Industrial and Engineering Chemistry* 19 (1927): 1202–1205; Frank O. Taylor, "Forty-five Years of Manufacturing Pharmacy," *Journal of the American Pharmaceutical Association* 4 (1915): 468–481. More scholarly is a study of the H. K. Mulford Company of Philadelphia, by Jonathan Liebenau, *Medical Science and Medical Industry: The Formation of the American Pharmaceutical Industry* (Baltimore: Johns Hopkins University Press, 1987). Also see John P. Swann, "The Evolution of the American Pharmaceutical Industry," *Pharmacy in History* 37 (1995): 76–86.

7. The term *ethical drug* today means one that is available only by prescription. Until 1997 it also meant the drug was not advertised to the public, but FDA rules have been relaxed to permit television and print advertising for certain categories of prescription medications. In the nineteenth century, *ethical* was applied to manufacturers who avoided popular publicity and who did not openly encourage self-medication. Their drugs might nevertheless be purchased by anyone who asked for them, with or without a prescription. Even after the turn of the century, a significant number of purchasers of ethical medicines were catalog merchants such as Sears, Roebuck, and Company and proprietors of rural general stores. Sears, for example, in 1900 carried laudanum at *USP* strength and a "French specific" for venereal disease. Sears, Roebuck and Co., *Fall Catalog, 1900* (reprint, Northfield, Ill.: Gun Digest Publishing, 1979), 14–27. See also Boris Emmet and John Jeuck, *Catalogues and Counters: A History of Sears, Roebuck and Company* (Chicago: University of Chicago Press, 1950), 248.

8. Robley Dunglison, *New Remedies: Pharmaceutically and Therapeutically Considered*, 4th ed., with extensive modifications and additions (Philadelphia: Lea and Blanchard, 1843), 446–453, 545–559.

9. See David L. Cowen, "The Role of the Pharmaceutical Industry," in *Safeguarding the Public: Historical Aspects of Medicinal Drug Control*, ed. J. L. Blake (Baltimore: Johns Hopkins University Press, 1970).

10. American Chemical Institute, *Positive Medical Agents: Being a Treatise on the New Alkaloid, Resinoid, and Concentrated Preparations of Indigenous and Foreign Medical Plants* (New York: Charles B. Norton, 1855), 18. The anonymous author then went on to say how dismayed he was by contemporary attacks on the integrity of physicians, but he also was aware that many doctors prescribed "without sufficiently inquiring into the causes which are operating on the system" (21).

11. L. Ausfield, "Turning over a New Leaf," *Druggists Circular* 33 (1889): 60.

12. The drug might eventually be discarded, but the key to the improvement of medical knowledge, said Parke-Davis, was for physicians to communicate their findings, whatever they were. "How to Test a New Drug," *Therapeutic Gazette* 6 (1882): 383–384. The *Gazette* was a Parke-Davis publication.

13. Cover advertisement, *New Preparations* 3 (1879), also a Parke-Davis publication.

14. Liebenau, *Medical Science and Medical Industry*, 34.

15. "Substitution of Drugs in Prescriptions by Druggists," *Medical Record* 29 (1886): 15.

16. "Like so many other aspects of the industry, this [intensive marketing] has been a post–World War II development." Walter S. Measday, "The Pharmaceutical Industry," in *The Structure of American Industry*, 5th ed., ed. Walter Adams (New York: Macmillan, 1977), 269.

17. On the late twentieth-century situation, see, for example, Joel Lexchin, *The Real Pushers: A Critical Analysis of the Canadian Drug Industry* (Vancouver: New Star Books, 1984); Milton M. Silberman and P. R. Lee, *Pills, Profits, and Politics* (Berkeley: University of California Press, 1974); John Braithwaite, *Corporate Crime in the Pharmaceutical Industry* (London: Routledge and Kegan Paul, 1984); letters to the editor regarding "Physicians and the Pharmaceutical Industry," *Annals of Internal Medicine* 113 (1990): 407–408; a position paper of the American College of Physicians, "Physicians and the Pharmaceutical Industry," *Annals of Internal Medicine* 112 (1990): 624–626; Harold Walton, "Ad Recognition and Prescribing by Physicians," *Journal of Advertising Research* 20 (1980): 39–48; R. B. Rand, "Pharmaceutical Advertising to Doctors," *Journal of Business* 14 (1941): 150–168; Pierre Garai, "Advertising and Promotion of Drugs," in *Drugs in Our Society*, ed. P. Talalay (Baltimore: Johns Hopkins University Press, 1964); Harry Dowling, "How Do Practicing Physicians Use New Drugs?" *JAMA* 185 (1963): 233–236; "Prescriptions for Profit," produced by Elizabeth Arledge, WGBH Educational Foundation, Boston, and originally broadcast 28 March 1989.

18. See John J. Black, *Forty Years in the Medical Profession, 1858–1898* (Philadelphia: Lippincott, 1900), 136ff.

19. "[The company] manifested that progressiveness and excellence in character of their products, for which they have been noted ever since"; R. F. Fairthorne, "Some Facts Concerning the Morphia and Opium Trade in the United States," *American Journal of Pharmacy* 52 (1880): 615. See also Tom Mahoney, *Merchants of Life: An Account of the American Pharmaceutical Industry* (New York: Harper and Brothers, 1959), esp. chap. 3; Liebenau, *Medical Science and Medical Industry*, chap. 2; George Urdang, "Retail Pharmacy as the Nucleus of the Pharmaceutical Industry," *Bulletin of the History of Medicine*, supp. 3 (1944): 325–346.

20. George Dohrmann III, "Medical Education in the United States as Seen by a German Immigrant: The Letters of George Dohrmann, 1897–1901," *Journal of the History of Medicine and Allied Sciences* 33 (1978): 477–506.

21. William Osler, *Aequanimitas* (London: H. K. Lewis, 1904), 301.

22. William G. Rothstein, *American Medical Schools and the Practice of Medicine: A History* (New York: Oxford University Press, 1987), 42.

23. An article in one journal, for example, told readers that the products of B. Keith and Company of New York "have proven, in every instance, all that is claimed for them." V. L. Hurlbut, "Concentrated Organic Medicines" *Medical Examiner* 1 (1860): 276–277.

24. Rarely did the names of any pharmaceutical companies appear in these articles unless it was a company-sponsored publication. So when a Kansas doctor wrote, "I instruct my druggist to specify P., D. & Co.'s preparations," we are not surprised to find it published in a Parke-Davis journal. J. L. Scott, "New Preparations," *New Preparations* 3 (1879): 11–12.

25. Pamela Walker Laird, "The Business of Progress: The Transformation of American Advertising, 1870–1920," 2 vols., Ph.D. dissertation, Boston University, 1992, esp. chap. 1.

26. Mahoney, *Merchants of Life*, 32.

27. Advertisement in *New York Medical Journal* 5 (1867). This was an "eclectic" firm, specializing in botanical preparations. The items were clearly presented as ingredients, however, not as "consumer-ready" concoctions. They were listed by their botanical or Latin names, and only two or three were mixtures rather than single entities.

28. Roscoe Rollins Clark, *Threescore Years and Ten: A Narrative of the First Seventy Years of Eli Lilly and Company, 1876–1946* (Indianapolis: privately published, 1946), 28.

29. Advertisement in *Medical and Surgical Reporter* 34 (1876).

30. Liebenau, *Medical Science and Medical Industry*, 18. In 1858 one editor commented negatively on some manufactured pills only because they were mislabeled. *Cincinnati Lancet-Observer*, n.s. 1 (1858): 694–696.

31. "Elegance in Prescribing," *Detroit Review of Medicine and Pharmacy* 5 (1870): 93–95.

32. James Harvey Young, *The Toadstool Millionaires: A Social History of Patent Medicine in America before Federal Regulation* (Princeton: Princeton University Press, 1961), chap. 1. These particular medicines were listed by their inventors' names in an advertisement for Garnier, Lamoureux and Co., Paris; *New York Medical Journal* 5 (1867).

33. The compound was for the treatment of exophthalmic goiter. The article in question had appeared in the January 1874 issue of the *Journal of Medical Science*. The advertisement appeared in *Northwestern Medical and Surgical Journal* 4 (1874).

34. Advertisements in *New York Medical Journal* 5 (1867). The rival company was Hegeman and Company of New York.

35. Advertisement in *Boston Medical and Surgical Journal* 90 (1874).

36. Advertisement for Hance Brothers of Philadelphia in *Northwestern Medical and Surgical Journal* 4 (1874).

37. Advertisement in *New York Medical Journal* 5 (1867).

38. Advertisement in *Medical and Surgical Reporter* 34 (1876).

39. The agents for a French manufacturer warned physicians that "They must be careful to see that the Pills dispensed by the Druggists are made by Messrs. Garnier, Lamoureux, & Co." Advertisement in *New York Medical Journal* 5 (1867).

40. Advertisement in *Boston Medical and Surgical Journal* 90 (1874).

41. Advertisement in *Cincinnati Lancet-Observer* 19 (1876).

42. Advertisement in *American Medical Gazette* 6 (1855). The elixir had been owned by the A.B. and D. Sands Company of New York City since 1841 but was evidently being imitated, so the company took pains to advise dealers and purchasers "that no Elixir of Opium [would] hereafter be genuine unless having their signature on the outside wrapper."

43. John S. Haller, "With a Spoonful of Sugar: The Art of Prescription Writing in the Late Nineteenth and Early Twentieth Century," *Pharmacy in History* 26 (1984): 171–178. Also see "The Importance of a Knowledge of the Physical Character of Drugs," *Boston Medical and Surgical Journal* 110 (1884): 595.

44. Parke-Davis advertisement in *Boston Medical and Surgical Journal* 90 (1874); Stearns ad in *Detroit Review of Medicine and Pharmacy* 11 (December 1876). This ad listed nineteen other botanical substances, placing each of them in a pharmacological category such as alterative, tonic, diuretic, and so forth. This may have been seen as merely practical, because the plants were not familiar ones, but the list also indicated the ailments for which each item was suitable. Woodruff ad in *JAMA* 19 (1892) December.

45. Advertisement in *Guardian of Health* 8 (April 1869). Stearns also had a copyrighted version of "purified opium," which, according to the ad, was preferable to the crude variety "for those compelled to use opium habitually." Years later, when he was reinstated in the APhA, Stearns expressed regret for his actions. Roland Lakey, "Frederick Stearns, Pharmacist," *Journal of the American Pharmaceutical Association (Practical Pharmacy Edition)* 9 (1948): 486–489.

46. *Ephemeris* 1 (1882): 145. *Ephemeris* was an occasional publication of the Squibb company. See also "An Enterprise Built upon Standardized Drugs," *Chemist and Druggist* 169 (1958): 635.

47. In 1888 a drug journal reported that Dr. Squibb was engaged in a "war on cascara" (Parke-Davis's popular laxative) because his own company dealt with a different botanical cathartic, and he was jealous of other's success. Moreover, the journal suggested Squibb had "achieved fame and fortune by overcharging for certain preparations like ether, chloroform, etc." The "only manufacturer who puts M.D. on all his labels and wares," Squibb had always been reputable, said the journal, but now he appeared foolish. He could not seem "to separate the interests of trade from those of progressive pharmacy." "Rhamnus vs Cascara," *Druggists Circular* 32 (1888): 1; "The Squibb Issue," *Druggists Circular* 32 (1888): 4–5. Nonetheless, few other manufacturers ever were held in as high regard. See Joseph Remington, "Edward Robinson Squibb, M.D.," *American Journal of Pharmacy* 73 (1901): 419–431.

48. Advertisement titled "The Relationship of Pharmacy to Medicine," *Buffalo Medical and Surgical Journal* 20 (June 1881).

49. Ibid.

50. Parke-Davis did not reject patents out of hand, however, having acquired one for a pill-making machine in 1888. Glenn Sonnedecker and George Griffenhagen, "A History of Sugar-Coated Pills and Tablets," *Journal of the American Pharmaceutical Association (Practical Pharmacy Edition)* 18 (1957): 486–489, 553–555.

51. Advertisement titled "Scientific and Business Platform," *Buffalo Medical and Surgical Journal* 33 (February 1894).

52. D. P. Duncan, "A Voice from the South on the Trade Mark Question," *Therapeutic Gazette* 6 (1882): 211.

53. Advertisement in *Southern Medical Journal* 12 (1919). The company was always proud of its record. For one thing, between 1885 and 1895, Parke-Davis paid for the annual publication of *Index Medicus*, which listed almost every article on medical subjects published anywhere in the world. See Taylor, "Forty-five Years of Manufacturing Pharmacy."

54. Chapter II, article I, section 4 of the 1847 Code of Ethics. David Dykstra analyzes in some detail the attitudes of practitioners to this class of drugs and the efforts of the AMA to educate its members and the profession at large to avoid them: Dykstra, "The Medical Profession and Patent and Proprietary Drugs during the Nineteenth Century," *Bulletin of the History of Medicine* 29 (1955): 401–419.

55. Full-page advertisement, *Cincinnati Lancet-Clinic*, n.s. 7 (1881). See Vincent Vinikas, *Soft Soap, Hard Sell: American Hygiene in an Age of Advertisement* (Ames: Iowa State University Press, 1992), esp. chap. 2, on how Listerine became a mouthwash.

56. C. A. Lindsley, "The Prescription of Proprietary Medicines for the Sick—Its Demoralizing Effects on the Medical Profession," *Therapeutic Gazette* 6 (1882): 361–368.

57. E. Eliot Harris, "Ethical Proprietary Preparations," *JAMA* 34 (1900): 1018.

58. "The Use of Proprietary Medicines," *Medical Record* 11 (1876): 423–424.

59. B. Joy Jeffries, "Re-establishment of the Medical Profession," *Boston Medical and Surgical Journal* 118 (1884): 589–593, 613–617. "In no country in the world are quacks more abundant than in the United States"; Francis J. Shepherd, "Medical Quacks and Quackery," *Popular Science Monthly* 23 (1883): 161.

60. Lindsley, "Proprietary Medicines," 362.

61. Ibid., 365.

62. This article was reprinted from the *Philadelphia Ledger*; "Medical Ethics and Business," *New York Times*, 22 April 1883, p. 14, col. 6.

63. J. H. Larkin, "The Influence of Proprietary Pharmacy upon the Practice of Medicine," *Boston Medical and Surgical Journal* 120 (1889): 11–15.

64. Emlen Painter, "The Medicines of Medicine," *Druggists Circular* 31 (1887): 257. The proprietary trade's own figures were far higher: 563 establishments in all

states; New York alone was home to 108. "Patent Medicine" *Boston Globe*, 17 August 1885, pp. 1, 2, 4.

65. Otto Wall, "Manufacturers' Preparations Ordered in Prescriptions," *Proceedings of the American Pharmaceutical Association* 32 (1884): 428–431, 540.

66. J. Marion Sims, "Anniversary Address before the American Medical Association," *Cincinnati Lancet-Observer* 19 (1876): 711–727.

67. "Dangerous Drug Preparations and the Duty of Journals Regarding Them," *Medical Science* 1 (1888): 228–230. The editor of the *Medical Record*, writing in a popular magazine, praised the "elegant and almost tasty compounds of modern pharmacy." George Shrady, "Recent Triumphs in Medicine and Surgery," *Forum* 23 (1897): 28–41.

68. R. O. Semmes, "The Medical Profession and the Medical Journals in Relation to Nostrums," *Boston Medical and Surgical Journal* 154 (1906): 331. Parke-Davis was pleased that its own record in this area could withstand scrutiny. The company had indeed enabled cascara sagrada and several other new items to receive trials and had undertaken to determine in what form these articles could be efficiently and safely manufactured. In 1879, Parke-Davis had also introduced a purified extract of ergot, "the first liquid extract to be standardized by chemical means," an important advance in botanical-source drugs notorious for their inconsistency. By 1883 it was offering other "normal liquids" as well, but the company never sought to patent any of them. *Parke Davis at 100* (Detroit: privately published, 1966), unpaginated.

69. "Should the Physician Prescribe Patented Drugs?" *JAMA* 33 (1899): 169; "Tablet-Triturates and Ready-Made Prescriptions," *JAMA* 34 (1900): 944–945.

70. "Dangerous Drug Preparations," 229.

71. N. Van Beil, "Adverse Legislation," *Druggists Circular* 33 (1889): 132.

72. Harry M. Archer, "The Wholesale Prescribing of Manufactured Medicines," *Medical Record* 37 (1890): 164.

73. "Close observation shows that there are few medical journals that can not be bribed into defrauding their readers in one way or another"; P. Maxwell Foshay, "Medical Ethics and Medical Journals," *JAMA* 34 (1900): 1041–1043.

74. Editorial, *Therapeutic Gazette* 6 (1882): 269–270. As part of its investigations of new drug products, Parke-Davis had promised to publish the results whether "good, bad or indifferent"; advertisement, *Buffalo Medical and Surgical Journal* 20 (June 1881). To do so, the company provided its own journal, *New Preparations* (established in 1877), renamed *The Therapeutic Gazette* in 1880. This publication had 5,000 regular readers but also distributed 20,000 free copies "with a view to bringing in returns in the way of actual subscribers." The journal appears to have been sensitive to the charge that it was merely a house organ. The editor reacted sarcastically to the Tilden Company's remarks about cascara sagrada (a Parke-Davis specialty); "The Ethical Combat," *New Preparations* 3 (1879): 16. The editor assured readers of the Parke-Davis journal that its pages would not

promote anything not meritorious; "The Aim and Object of *New Preparations*," *New Preparations* 3 (1879): 228–230.

75. "Advertisements," *JAMA* 1 (1883): 89; G. R. Henry, letter to the editor, *JAMA* 1 (1883): 93–94. Parke-Davis also aroused the ire of the *Pharmaceutical Era*, an independent Detroit journal. Although the journal does not provide details, the company's behavior compelled the *Era* to renew its advertising contract with Parke-Davis at a rate 50 percent higher than that of the previous year. "This is a polite way which publishers sometimes have of telling a firm that they do not care for their business. . . . We have declined their business, and they know very well that we do not solicit or desire their patronage"; *Pharmaceutical Era* 10 (1893): 339.

76. Long before *JAMA*, the advertising price list of the *Northwestern Medical and Surgical Journal* of St. Paul, Minnesota (1871, vol. 2) made this claim, which may have led to conflict between the editor and the publishers. Alexander J. Stone, M.D., the first editor of this journal (1870), appended some remarks to the advertising price list that appeared in December 1871. Advertisements, he said, were the responsibility of the publisher, implying that he, the editor, could not always control the quality or the kind of advertising being accepted. Stone was removed as of June 1872, and the publishers edited the journal themselves. Insufficient material remains to judge whether the new editors increased the number of advertising pages.

77. "Advertisements," *Cincinnati Lancet-Clinic* 8 (1882): 292.

78. William C. Alpers, "Prescription Repetition and Its Dangers," *JAMA* 40 (1903): 1078–1080.

79. M. Clayton Thrush, "Modern Prescribing," *Pharmaceutical Era* 33 (1905): 70–72.

80. Charles S. Williamson, "The Responsibility of the Medical Teacher for Existing Conditions," *JAMA* 46 (1900): 1342–1344; N. S. Davis, "Effect of Proprietary Literature on Medical Men," *JAMA* 46 (1906): 1338–1339; Robert Hessler, "A Study of Proprietary Medicine Advertisements," *JAMA* 44 (1905): 1982–1986. An Ohio doctor, for example, when attempting to evaluate a new type of preparation, said he wanted an "honest assessment," not one provided by the manufacturers. S. Herbert Britton, "Guaiacol," *Cincinnati Lancet-Clinic* 40 (1898): 392–394. Another physician was distressed that proprietary prescribing "put money into the pockets of those who . . . have wantonly departed from the noble rule of our clan, that whatever the individual finds and proves to be of merit belongs to the profession, not to the discoverer alone." A.K.P. Meserve, "The Use of Advertised Drugs by Physicians, " *Journal of Medicine and Science* 4 (1897–1898): 271–277; G. B. Kuykendall, "Relation of Physicians to the So-called 'Ethical' Proprietary Medicines," *JAMA* 46 (1906): 1992–1993; Joseph Pettit, "The Evils of Proprietary Medicines," *JAMA* 46 (1906): 402–405.

81. G. Frank Lydston, "Medicine as a Business Proposition," *JAMA* 34 (1900): 1316–1321, 1400–1404.

82. J. F. Beery, "The Proper Place for Proprietaries," *JAMA* 33 (1899): 896–898. J. H. Salisbury, "The Subordination of Medical Journals to Proprietary Interests,"

JAMA 46 (1906): 1337–1338. The *Cincinnati Lancet-Clinic*, however, wanted it made clear that the "proprietary" medicines advertised in its pages were not the same as "patent" medicines, the latter often being of "the prurient kind." A reader responded tartly that "fraudulent advertisements [were] not always filthy, nor [were] religious or other papers the only dupes," but all proprietary drugs were the same in their duplicity. The *Lancet*'s ethical standing, he said, was at risk. D. R. Silver, "The Patent Medicine Crusade," *Cincinnati Lancet-Clinic* 94 (1905): 675–676.

83.   "The U.S. Pharmacopoeia and New Drugs," *American Medical Quarterly* 1 (1899): 183–185. It is therefore rather ironic that this journal included any number of "articles" about the merits of the very drugs found on its advertising pages. Most of these items were on the reformers' list of unprofessional medicines.

84.   Davis, "Effect of Proprietary Literature."

85.   Why trust the manufacturer? asked one Buffalo pharmacist-physician. Go to the *USP* instead. Charles Abbott, "The Evils Attending the Wholesale Administration of Drugs in Tablet Form," *American Medicine* 6 (1903): 262; John Ritter, "Pharmacopeia or Proprietary Prescriptions: Which?" *JAMA* 47 (1906): 683–684. Science would help practitioners better evaluate the options: John Aulde, "The Basis of Scientific Therapeutics," *American Therapist* 1 (1892): 101–104; John Billings, "Ideals of Medical Education" *Science* 18 (1891): 1–4, 15–17.

86.   Daniel Webster Cathell, *Book on the Physician Himself and Things That Concern His Reputation and Success*, 10th ed. (Philadelphia: F. A. Davis Co., 1898), 276. Cathell also preferred ambiguous explanations so that patients would not become too well informed and simply collude with the pharmacist the next time they needed treatment.

CHAPTER 4   THE REMARKABLE SYNTHETIC DRUGS

1.   For an excellent account, see Anthony S. Travis, *The Rainbow Makers: The Origins of the Synthetic Dyestuffs Industry in Western Europe* (Bethlehem, Pa.: Lehigh University Press, 1993).

2.   For an interesting contemporary account, see Charlton Bastian et al., "Discussion of the Germ Theory of Disease," *Transactions of the Pathological Society of London* 26 (1875): 255–345.

3.   James T. Whittaker, "Doctrines of Therapy," *Cincinnati Lancet-Clinic*, n.s. 15 (1885): 551–559. See also William H. Draper, "The Principles and Progress of Modern Therapeutics," *Medical Record* 30 (1886): 589–593. Once associated with quacks and empirics, specificity was now taking on a decidedly legitimate cast.

4.   John K. Crellin, "Internal Antisepsis or the Dawn of Chemotherapy?" *Journal of the History of Medicine and Allied Sciences* 36 (1981): 9–18.

5.   See G. June Goodfield, *The Growth of Scientific Physiology* (London: Hutchinson, 1960); Everett Mendelsohn, *Heat and Life: The Development of the Theory of Animal*

Heat (Cambridge: Harvard University Press, 1964). Both authors argue the importance of "heat" as a concept central to physiological thought.

6. Charles E. Rosenberg, "The Tyranny of Diagnosis: Specific Entities and Individual Experience," *Milbank Quarterly* 80 (2002): 242.

7. Jan McTavish, "Antipyretic Treatment and Typhoid Fever, 1860–1900," *Journal of the History of Medicine and Allied Sciences* 42 (1987): 486–506.

8. Not until the 1890s were the causative organisms of malaria identified and quinine's real mode of action discovered. Gordon Harrison, *Mosquitoes, Malaria and Man: A History of the Hostilities since 1880* (London: John Murray, 1978), 11–12.

9. One of the best contemporary summaries of fever research can be found in Paul Joseph Lorain, *De la température du corps humain et de ses variations dans les diverses maladies*, 2 vols. (Paris: Imprimerie Nationale, 1877).

10. A summary of antipyretic therapies can be found in Silvio Rageth, "Die antipyretische Welle in der zweiten Hälfte des 19. Jahrhunderts," *Zürcher Medizingeschichtliche Abhandlungen*, n. s. 24 (1964).

11. See John J. Beer, *The Emergence of the German Dye Industry* (Urbana: University of Illinois Press, 1959); he discusses patents on p. 105. Aaron Ihde, *The Development of Modern Chemistry* (New York: Harper and Row, 1964), chap. 17; Fritz L. Haber, *The Chemical Industry during the Nineteenth Century* (Oxford: Oxford University Press, 1958); W. Gardner, ed., *The British Coal Tar Industry* (London: Williams and Norgate, 1915); P. M. Hohenberg, *Chemicals in Western Europe, 1850–1914: An Economic Study of Technical Change* (Chicago: Rand McNally, 1967). Also see Chartered Institute of Patent Agents, *Patent Laws of the World*, 4th ed., 2 vols. (London, 1911).

12. See Thomas M. Reimer, "Bayer and Company in the United States: German Dyes, Drugs and Cartels in the Progressive Era," Ph.D. dissertation, Syracuse University, 1996; in chap. 1 he deals with the German background. Also instructive about the patent situation (because it records rejected applications, including items eventually awarded patents in other countries) is Adolf Winther, *Zusammenstellung der Patente auf dem Gebiete der organischen Chemie 1877 bis 1905*, 3 vols. (Giessen: A. Töppelmann, 1908–1910).

13. See Georg Meyer-Thurow, "The Industrialization of Invention: A Case Study from the German Chemical Industry," *Isis* 73 (1982): 363–381; Timothy Lenoir, "A Magic Bullet: Research for Profit and the Growth of Knowledge in Germany around 1900," *Minerva* 26 (1988): 66–88; Jonathan Liebenau, "Paul Ehrlich as a Commercial Scientist and Research Administrator," *Medical History* 34 (1990): 65–78.

14. Hermann Kolbe, "Über eine neue Darstellungsmethode und einige bemerkenswerthe Eigenschaften der Salicylsäure," *Journal für Praktische Chemie*, n. s. 18 (1874): 89–112. Kolbe and a colleague had actually synthesized salicylic acid in 1859 but had not exploited the discovery at that time.

15. Salicylic acid itself had first been isolated in the early 1800s but had rarely been

used in medicine. A related substance, salicin, had also been isolated early in the century and had found use as a substitute for cinchona and quinine, although it too never achieved much popularity. Most modern commentators on the salicylates consider that because these chemicals can be found in nature (the English *salicylate* being derived from *salix*, the Latin word for willow) and were used by healers in antiquity, their use as analgesics and antipyretics stretches back to Hippocrates. I, however, can find no reference in the work of any ancient author that unequivocally describes these attributes of salicylate-bearing plants. Hippocrates, for example, used willow leaf *smoke* as a postpartum uterine fumigant, not as an analgesic in childbirth, as is frequently claimed. See Hippocrates, "Des malades des femmes," in *Ouevres completes*, trans. and ed. Emil Littré, 10 vols. (Paris: Buillière, 1839–1861), 8:187. See also Edward Stone, "An Account of the Success of the Bark of the Willow in the Cure of Agues," *Philosophical Transactions of the Royal Society* 53 (1763): 195–200. Reverend Stone remarked on the fact that willow was not used much, but his suggestion that it could be a cheap substitute for cinchona was not taken up.

16. See Dr. Stricker, "Über die Resultate der Behandlung der Polyarthritis rheumatica mit Salicylsäure," *Berliner Klinische Wochenschrift* 13 (1876): 1–2, 15–16. "Quickly" usually meant within one to three days. A. Clark, "Salicylate of Soda in Rheumatism," *Medical Record* 11 (1876): 663–665.

17. See the bibliography in A. Geissler, "Über die antipyretische Wirkung der Salicylsäure und der salicylsauren Salze," *Jahrbücher der in-und ausländischen gesammten Medicin* 172 (1876): 185–202.

18. *Scientific American*, May 1880, reprinted in *Scientific American* 242 (1980): 13. Kolbe himself thought the acid could do no wrong: Alan J. Rocke, *The Quiet Revolution: Hermann Kolbe and the Science of Organic Chemistry* (Berkeley: University of California Press, 1993), 304–309.

19. Rocke, *Quiet Revolution*, 306.

20. "Secrets of the Druggists," *New York Times*, 11 June 1882, p. 10, cols. 4–5.

21. "Salicin and salicylic acid are unquestionably among the most valuable articles in our materia medica, but for all this they are *drugs*, and all drugs must be handled cautiously, else they are potent for harm"; "A Therapeutic Warning," *Druggists Circular* 27 (1883): 166 (emphasis in original).

22. Ernst Bäumler has published several works on the history of Hoechst: *A Century of Chemistry*, trans. D. Goodman (Dusseldorf: Econ Verlag, 1968); *Die Rotfabriker: Familiengeschichte eines Weltunternehmens* (Munich: Piper, 1988); and *Farben, Formeln, Forscher: Hoechst und die Geschichte der industriellen Chemie in Deutschland* (Munich: Piper, 1989). See also Hermann Pinnow, *Zur Erinnerung an die 75: Wiederkehr des Gründungstages der Farbwerke vorm: Meister Lucius und Bruning* (Munich: F. Bruckmann, 1938).

23. Wilhelm Filehne, "Über neue Mittel, welche die fieberhafte Temperatur zur Norm bringen," *Berliner Klinische Wochenschrift* 19 (1882): 681–683; Wilhelm Filehne, "Weiteres über Kairin und analoge Körper," *Berliner Klinische*

Wochenschrift 20 (1883): 77–79. See also K. Brune, "Knorr and Filehne in Erlangen," in *One Hundred Years of Pyrazolone Drugs: An Update*, ed. K. Brune (Basel: Birkhäuser Verlag, 1986), 28.

24. Beverley Robinson, "Some Critical Remarks in Regard to the Use of Antipyretic Agents in Typhoid Fever," *New York Medical Journal* 37 (1883): 574–576. Robinson found Kairin too dangerous and advised caution.

25. G.H.C. Klie, "Kairin," *Druggists Circular* 27 (1883): 179–180; quinine sulphate in this period cost about sixty to seventy-five cents per ounce (one ounce weighs 28 grams). Despite its drawbacks, Hoechst did not give up production. Kairin remained available for many years and presumably found some uses.

26. See Harry M. Marks, *The Progress of Experiment: Science and Therapeutic Reform in the United States, 1900–1990* (Cambridge: Cambridge University Press, 1997), chap. 1, which provides a short, useful summary of the late nineteenth-century situation. Charles E. Rosenberg, "The Therapeutic Revolution: Medicine, Meaning, and Social Change in Nineteenth-Century America," in *The Therapeutic Revolution: Essays in the Social History of American Medicine*, ed. Morris J. Vogel and Charles E. Rosenberg (Philadelphia: University of Pennsylvania Press, 1979); John Harley Warner, "Ideals of Science and Their Discontents in Late Nineteenth-Century American Medicine," *Isis* 82 (1981): 454–478. See also K. Codell Carter, "The Development of Pasteur's Concept of Disease Causation and the Emergence of Specific Causes in Nineteenth-Century Medicine," *Bulletin of the History of Medicine* 65 (1991): 528–548.

27. Despite claims that therapies were based on scientific theories, chemical and pharmacological studies in the nineteenth century tended to be performed well after a drug had been extensively employed clinically. Other sorts of investigations might only be performed by accident—as in the case of a woman in her ninth month of pregnancy who went into premature labor after her physician gave her Antipyrine for a fever. Wondering whether the drug had been the cause, the doctor gave sixty grains in divided doses to twelve pregnant patients. None of them went into early labor. (He did not state if the women knew they were involved in an experiment.) "The Non-Injurious Effect of Antipyrine in Pregnancy," *Medical News* 47 (1885): 132. Even in the early twentieth century, orthodox medicine was really just "crude empiricism at its very worst" when it came to evaluating medications, according to Frederic S. Lee, "The Relation of the Medical Sciences to Clinical Medicine," *Columbia University Quarterly* 17 (1914–1915): 127–142.

28. An account of Antipyrine's discovery, as well as references to virtually every article ever published on the drug up to 1950, can be found in Leon A. Greenberg, *Antipyrine: A Critical Bibliographic Review* (New Haven, Conn.: Hillhouse Press, 1950).

29. Culbertson seems to be an ideal sort of physician, reading widely and even doing his own clinical trials, but how typical he was is difficult to determine.

Howard Culbertson, "Antipyrine and Its Uses," *Cincinnati Lancet-Clinic* 16 (1886): 251–255.

30. A. C. Girard, "Antipyrin—The New Antipyretic," *Medical News* 45 (1884): 625–627.

31. "Antipyrin," *Druggists Circular* 28 (1884): 185.

32. "Antipyrine a Substitute for Quinine," *New York Times*, 1 January 1886, p. 6, col. 4. Newspapers were becoming one of the avenues by which information about new drugs reached large numbers of the public, a situation the AMA was not happy with: "Mania for Novelties in Medicine," *JAMA* 8 (1887): 549; Henry Smith Williams, "The Century's Progress in Scientific Medicine," *Harper's Magazine* 99 (1899): 38–52. Terra Ziporyn has noted that the public was only interested if scientific medicine suggested possible treatments and cures, not merely curious facts: Ziporyn, *Disease in the Popular American Press: The Case of Diphtheria, Typhoid Fever, and Syphilis, 1870–1920* (New York: Greenwood Press, 1988). See also Hyman Kuritz, "The Popularization of Science in Nineteenth-Century America," *History of Education Quarterly* 21 (1981): 259–274. Kuritz links the increasing interest in science to the growing secularization of American society.

Antipyrine was also credited as effective in treating epilepsy, whooping cough, chorea, seasickness, and many other conditions; wishful thinking surpassed reality, and this medication was sometimes in danger of becoming yet another disappointing panacea. See, for example, "Some of the Less Common Uses of Antipyrine," *Medical Record* 31 (1887): 242; William H. German, "Some of the Uses of Antipyrin," *Medical Record* 33 (1888): 68.

33. A. Cahn and P. Hepp, "Das Antifebrin, ein neues Fiebermittel," *Centralblatt für Klinische Medicin* 7 (1886): 561–564. For the story of the drug's apparently accidental discovery, see Martin Gross, *Acetanilid: A Critical Bibliographic Review* (New Haven, Conn.: Hillhouse Press, 1946): 1–3. More recent scholars, however, say the story is probably not true and seems to have arisen in the 1920s, although no one knows why. See Laurie Prescott, *Paracetamol (Acetaminophen): A Critical Bibliographic Review* (London: Taylor and Francis, 1996), 1.

34. It is worth noting that Bayer's product was inspired by two things: Antifebrin's (acetanilid's) success and the fact that a waste material taking up space in Bayer's cellar could be converted into the similar chemical acetphenetidin, which the company then called Phenacetin. Carl Duisberg, "Zur Geschichte der Entdeckung des Phenacetins," in *Abhandlungen, Vorträge, und Reden aus den Jahren, 1882–1921* (Berlin: Verlag Chemie, 1923). Duisberg later became a director of Bayer and a prominent leader of the German chemical industry. Henry Armstrong, "The Chemical Industry and Carl Duisberg," *Nature* 135 (1935): 1021–1025. Paul K. Smith, *Acetophenetidin: A Critical Bibliographic Review* (New York: Interscience, 1958).

35. William Osler, "Antifebrin," *Transactions of the College of Physicians of Philadelphia* 9 (1887): 117–118, 119–121 (discussion). For physicians whose patients were poor, living in tenements, and caring for children, who could not stay in bed, eat well,

or travel for their health ("luxuries . . . as unattainable as a steam yacht"), the new drugs provided "artificial rest" without the dangers of opium. William F. Hutchinson, "Phenacetin in the Nervous Sequelae of La Grippe," *American Therapist* 1 (1892): 12.

36. Turning "intensely blue . . . may not have any serious consequences [but] it is certainly not agreeable to a sick person. . . . The blueness would be exceedingly apt to extend from the patient to the physician, especially if a suit for malpractice were instituted"; "Antifebrin," *Medical World* 4 (1886): 365. As alternatives to the synthetics, a Texas doctor offered his own antipyretic mixtures, all containing ipecac and quinine, but because they were difficult concoctions for a druggist or physician to make, he was hopeful that a manufacturer might be interested in producing them. B. Frank Humphreys, "Antipyretic Pills," *Therapeutic Gazette* 11 (1887): 746–747.

37. The chemical could be made by any reasonably equipped pharmacy, according to one observer, but appears at this time to have been almost exclusively a factory product made in Europe. F. J. Wulling, "Acetanilid, Antifebrin: How Prepared," *Pharmaceutical Era* 10 (1893): 397.

38. "The Free Advertising of New Foreign Drugs," *Boston Medical and Surgical Journal* 118 (1888): 637–638; reprint of *National Druggist* editorial.

39. "A New Antipyretic," *Boston Medical and Surgical Journal* 111 (1884): 162.

40. "Being prepared under the control of the most competent chemists, [Antipyrine] was not likely to vary in quality," noted the *American Druggist* 14 (1885): 162. Natural source drugs, on the other hand, could vary widely—one of their drawbacks. The professor of materia medica at the University of Pennsylvania agreed that Antipyrine deserved a patent for being an ingenious artificial item. Horatio C. Wood, "Nostrums," *JAMA* 32 (1899): 908–911. See also "Is It Proper for a Physician to Employ a Patented Drug?" *Medical News* 75 (1899): 46–47. The answer was yes, if the patent was the only proprietary feature it had.

41. "Antipyrin: The Newest Antipyretic," *Medical News* 45 (1884): 128–129.

42. J. Pfeiffer, "What Legislation Can Be Proposed to Check the Exorbitant Charges Made in This Country, by Foreign Manufacturers, on the So-called Patented Chemicals, as Compared with Prices Asked in Other Countries?" *Pharmaceutical Era* 21 (1899): 758. Pfeiffer's example was Aristol (thymol iodide), a Bayer product that cost 180 marks per kilo in Germany (where it was patented), 33 marks in Switzerland (no patent), and the equivalent of 237 marks in the United States.

43. Arthur Acheson, *Trade-Mark Advertising as an Investment* (New York: New York Evening Post, 1917), 46ff. See also Berthold Singer, *Trade Mark Laws of the World and Unfair Trade* (Chicago: Hammond Press, 1913.)

44. Julius Stieglitz, "The Problem of the Synthetic Chemical Compound," *JAMA* 46 (1906): 1341–1342. By the time Stieglitz was writing, the number of new synthetic products had risen dramatically, making the problem of learning their names even more difficult.

45. Kay Brune, quoting Filehne, in "Knorr and Filehne in Erlangen," 21; see also Elmar Ernst, *Das "industrielle" Geheimmittel und seine Werbung: Arzneifertigwaren in der zweiten Hälfte des 19: Jahrhunderts in Deutschland* (Würzburg: Jal-Verlag, 1975), 156.

46. See Samuel S. Adams, "Antipyrin; Its History, Physiological Action, and Therapeutic Effects," *JAMA* 5 (1885): 621–625.

47. Ludwig Knorr, "Einwirkung von Acetessigester auf Hydrazinchinizinderivate," *Berichte der Deutschen Chemischen Gesellschaft* 17 (1884): 546–552.

48. Ludwig Knorr, "Ueber die Constitution der Chinizinderivate," *Berichte der Deutschen Chemischen Gesellschaft* 17 (1884): 2032–2049.

49. Adolf Winther, *Zusammenstellung der Patent aus dem Gebiete der organischen Chemie* (Giessen: A. Töppelmann, 1877–1905), 1:1134.

50. George B. Shattuck, "The Results of the Use of Antipyrine at the Boston City Hospital," *Boston Medical and Surgical Journal* 113 (1885): 78–80. Shattuck had reported on Kairin in 1883, when he had anticipated correctly that a better drug would be found: Kairin had already passed out of use.

51. In the 1890s, Hoechst developed Pyramidon (aminopyrine), an analgesic antipyretic that appears to have remained largely a professional drug and did not become particularly popular with the laity, although it was reportedly a very powerful analgesic. It was recognized as being quite toxic, and its use in the United States and some other countries has been discontinued.

52. George N. Acker, "Notes on the Use of Antipyrine in Fevers," *JAMA* 5 (1885): 571–572, 581 (discussion).

53. "Not *Antifibrin*, but *Antifebrin*," *American Druggist* 16 (1887): 155–156.

54. "Another New Antipyretic—Antifebrin," *Medical Record* 30 (1886): 294.

55. In 1887 a Chicago wholesale druggist, for example, listed both acetanilid and Antifebrin at twenty-five cents per ounce, comparable to the prices of the drugs in Germany. (Antipyrine was $1.38; prices are those listed in *American Druggist* 15 [1886].) The W. H. Schieffelin Company of New York did not list acetanilid, but the "Antifebrine" it sold at twenty-five cents was noted as being of Kalle's manufacture. Peter van Schaak, another Chicago dealer, also sold acetanilid for twenty-five cents but Antifebrin for forty-five cents. (Antipyrine was $1.40.) In 1888, Schaak's price for Antifebrin came down to a more competitive twenty-five cents; acetanilid was now fifteen cents per ounce. By the end of the century it was listed at around eight cents per ounce or less, with the brand-name product at about twice that. Price books, Kremers Reference Files, University of Wisconsin, Madison.

56. Lyman F. Kebler, "Phenacetin: History, Patent, Methods of Manufacture and Chemical Constitution," *Proceedings of the American Pharmaceutical Association* 51 (1903): 365–377.

57. The prescription book of E. B. Heimstreet of Janesville, Wisconsin, for 1893–1894, contains quite a number of prescriptions for "phenacetin," some for

"Phenacetine Bayer," but none for "acetphenetidin"; file C39q, Kremers Reference Files.

58. John Blake White, "Antipyrin as an Analgesic in Headache," *Medical Record* 30 (1886): 293. He had studied the drug for two years before publishing his findings.

59. P. R. Egan, "Antipyrin as an Analgesic," *Medical Record* 34 (1888): 477–478. The names of these drugs are spelled with or without the final *e* throughout their histories.

60. F. Tuckerman, "Antipyrine in Cephalalgia," *Medical Record* (1888): 180.

61. W. H. Thomson addressing the New York Academy of Medicine, *New York Medical Journal* 46 (1887): 109.

62. William F. Wright, "The Uses of Antipyrin Other Than as an Antipyretic," *Medical Record* 32 (1887): 814.

63. T. S. Robertson, "Antipyrine in Migraine, Pyrexia, Etc.," *Medical Record* 31 (1887): 517–518. Robertson actually calls some of his patients neurotic, but it should be noted that in this period the term meant "related to the nerves."

64. Eustace L. Fiske, "Antipyrine as an Analgesic," *Boston Medical and Surgical Journal* 119 (1888): 34. See also the editorial "Antipyrine as an Analgesic," *Boston Medical and Surgical Journal* 116 (1887): 534–535. Another practitioner, however, thought that all the synthetics had "well-grounded claims to be rivals to opium." J.F.A. Adams, "Substitutes for Opium in Chronic Diseases," *Boston Medical and Surgical Journal* 121 (1889): 353.

65. Walther Faust, "Antifebrin gegen Kopfschmerz," *Deutsche Medizinische Wochenschrift* 13 (1887): 575.

66. Harvey B. Bashore, "Antifebrin in the Treatment of Headaches," *Medical Record* 36 (1889): 430–431.

67. J.M.G. Carter, "Use of Antipyrin and Antifebrin for Headaches," *JAMA* 11 (1888): 198–197.

68. F. T. Simpson, "Some Notes on Antifebrin," *Medical Record* 32 (1887): 706–707.

69. See also Alan M. Hamilton, "Antipyrine and Acetanilide (Antifebrin) in Headache and Epilepsy," *New York Medical Journal* 45 (1887): 593–594; Graeme Hammond, "Antipyrine for the Relief of Headaches," *Journal of Nervous and Mental Disease* 19 (1892): 282–285; R. R. Ball, "Antipyrine in Neuralgic Headache," *Medical Record* 33 (1888): 39.

70. A *Medical News* editorial (54 [1889]: 130) that had commented on Phenacetin's failure as an antipyretic had instead found the drug to be a good analgesic. The history of the drug as an analgesic is summarized in Smith, *Acetophenetidin*, chap. 7.

71. Hugo Hoppe, "Ueber die Wirkung des Phenacetins (Para-Acetphenetidin)," *Therapeutische Monatsheft* 2 (1888): 160–168.

72. Robertson, "Antipyrine in Migraine, Pyrexia, Etc."

73. All the aniline derivatives have toxic features, including kidney damage (Phenacetin) and potentially fatal blood disorders (acetanilid, Antipyrine, and especially Pyramidon), despite claims from the manufacturers even today that the dangers are highly exaggerated. See Brune, *One Hundred Years of Pyrazolone Drugs*. As for the side effects noted when the drugs were first introduced in the nineteenth century (cardiac problems and "collapse"), the authors of the *Critical Bibliographies* (Smith on Phenacetin, in *Acetophenetidin*, chap. 10; Gross on acetanilid, in *Acetanilid*, chap. 6; Greenberg on Antipyrine, in *Antipyrine*, chap. 6) examined all the published reports and concluded that most alleged fatalities either never occurred or could be attributed to other causes. Allergic reactions were not uncommon, however, and overdoses still produced untoward effects. By the 1970s, all of these drugs had been deleted from the American pharmacopeia, although they are still used in some other countries.

74. For example, T. W. Luce, "The Acetanilid Habit: Report of Two Cases," *American Medicine* 6 (1903): 502; "Antipyrin Habit," *Medical Record* 36 (1889): 700.

75. Even neurology, one of the newer medical sciences, could not accommodate painkilling: "The methods of pain control and treatment introduced in the mid-nineteenth century were difficult to reconcile" with theories of nerve action that had resulted from physiological investigations in France and Germany. Lawrence Kruger and Sandra Kroin, "A Brief Historical Survey of Concepts in Pain Research," in *Handbook of Perception*, ed. Edward Carterette and Morton Friedman (New York: Academic Press, 1978), 172.

76. Some physicians did identify the synthetics as primarily analgesic, although they did not endorse their use for most headaches. See Wharton Sinkler, "The Therapeutic Status of the Coal-Tar Products in Neuralgia and other Painful Conditions," *Therapeutic Gazette* 27 (1902): 4–6. Textbooks and other reference works, however, continued to catalog the drugs as antipyretics, with analgesia as a secondary property, to be employed only in limited circumstances.

77. Joseph Collins, "A Contribution to the Study of Headaches, with Particular Reference to Their Etiology and Treatment," *Medical Record* 41 (1892): 370–373.

78. James W. Putnam, "Headache," *JAMA* 21 (1893): 185–187.

79. Charles Graef, "Headaches of Ocular and Nasal Origin," *Medical Record* 75 (1909): 11–13. Graef was an ophthalmologist at Fordham University.

80. H. Gradle, "Diagnostic Characteristics of Headaches According to Their Origin," *JAMA* 31 (1898): 1222–1223.

81. G. P. Hachenberg, *Medical Consultation Book* (Austin: Eugene v. Boeckmann, 1893), 412–419.

82. Justin Herold, "The Treatment of Headache," *Boston Medical and Surgical Journal* 174 (1916): 15–17.

83. John Donovan, "Headache and Its Cures," *New York Medical Journal* 88 (1908): 310–311. Donovan nevertheless preferred laxatives and tonics.

84. Floyd Crego, "Treatment of Headache," *Buffalo Medical Journal* 35 (1895): 369–379. Exalgin was an American proprietary consisting of methyl acetanilid.

85. Daniel Clark, "Headache," *Canadian Practitioner* 19 (1894): 359–366. Clark also recommended that these "seductive" painkillers be disguised so that the patient would not self-medicate.

86. E. Castelli, "The Clinical Significance of the Symptom, Headache," *Medical Record* 72 (1907): 515–517.

87. Representatives of the headache literature after the turn of the century include J. Vernon White, "Headache," *Detroit Medical Journal* 4 (1904): 65–69; Gustaf Norstrom, "Chronic Headache and Its Treatment by Massage," *New York Medical Journal* 82 (1905): 956–962, 1008–1011, 1060–1063; S.W.S. Toms, "The Relation of Eye-Strain to Chronic Headaches," *JAMA* 48 (1907): 1009–1010; Samuel Stalberg, "Treatment of Sick Headache," *New York Medical Journal* 88 (1908): 1038–1039; Theodore Diller, "Chronic Constitutional Headaches," *International Clinics* 3 (1909): 259–270; Siegmund Auerbach, *Headache: Its Varieties, Their Nature, Recognition and Treatment* (London: Playfair, 1913). Almost every publication on the headache in this period stated very clearly that doctors should always establish the correct diagnosis before initiating treatment.

88. Woods Hutchinson, "The Value of Pain," *Monist* 7 (1896–1897): 494–504.

89. H. M. Whelpley, "Fashionable Medicines," *Druggists Circular* 33 (1889): 244.

CHAPTER 5   DRUGGISTS, DOCTORS, AND THE LAW

1. Glenn Sonnedecker, ed., *Kremers and Urdang's History of Pharmacy*, 4th ed. (Philadelphia: Lippincott, 1976), 157.

2. Advertisement for Henry White's drugstore, *Boston Medical Intelligencer* 4 (1827): 360.

3. Cover advertisement for C. D. Griswold of New York City, *Annalist: A Record of Practical Medicine in the City of New York* 1 (April 1847).

4. The Philadelphia College of Apothecaries was founded in 1821 as both a school and professional association, and was the model for subsequent institutions (Sonnedecker, *History of Pharmacy*, 190–192). See also Samuel Jackson, "On the Conditions of the Medicines of the United States—and the Means of Their Reform: An Introductory Lecture Delivered at the Philadelphia College of Pharmacy," *Philadelphia Journal of Medical and Physical Sciences* 5 (1822): 210–226.

5. Sonnedecker, *History of Pharmacy*, 198ff.

6. Charles LaWall, "Pharmaceutical Ethics," *Journal of the American Pharmaceutical Association* 10 (1921): 895–910. La Wall's anniversary discussion includes an account of the 1852 code.

7. See Lee Anderson and Gregory Higby, *The Spirit of Voluntarism: A Legacy of Commitment and Contribution: The "United States Pharmacopoeia," 1820–1995* (Rockville, Md.: United States Pharmacopeial Convention, 1995); Glenn

Sonnedecker, "Contributions of the Pharmaceutical Profession toward Controlling the Quality of Drugs in the Nineteenth Century," in *Safeguarding the Public: Historical Aspects of Medicinal Drug Control*, ed. J. B. Blake (Baltimore: Johns Hopkins University Press, 1970); Glenn Sonnedecker, "The *Pharmacopeia* and America—150 Years of Service," *Pharmacy in History* 12 (1970): 156–169. See also the series of articles by Glenn Sonnedecker, "The Founding Period of the *U.S. Pharmacopeia*," *Pharmacy in History* 35 (1993): 151–162; 36 (1994): 3–25, 103–122. On the legal status of pharmacy, see David Cowen, "The Development of State Pharmaceutical Law," *Pharmacy in History* 37 (1995): 49–58. Although the *USP* is "official," it was and has remained a private initiative, completely nongovernmental.

8. William Procter, Jr., "Thoughts on 'Manufacturing Pharmacy' in Its Bearing on the Practice of Pharmacy, and the Character and Qualifications of Pharmaceutists," *Druggists Circular* 2 (1858): 55.

9. Advertisement for Pond and Morse of Rutland, Vt., *Northern Lancet* 2 (1852).

10. Mahlon N. Kline, "Proprietary Preparations and the Retail Trade," *Druggists Circular* 34 (1890): 152. Kline did note that "the average druggist purchases at least nine tenths of his fluid extracts, and a large proportion of elixirs, but a very small proportion of his tinctures, wines, syrups, and preparations of that character." In 1891 the firm became the Smith, Kline and French Company.

11. E. N. Gathercoal, *The Prescription Ingredient Survey* (Chicago: American Pharmaceutical Association, 1933), 8. In Sussex County, N.J., by 1897 doctors were prescribing by brand name, according to one analysis of prescription records. Cyrus Ettinger, "Prescriptions: Circa 1872–1913," undated typescript, file C39q, Kremers Reference Files, University of Wisconsin, Madison.

12. Emlen Painter, "The Medicines of Medicine," *Druggists Circular* 31 (1887): 257.

13. "Physician and Pharmacist," *Medical Record* 18 (1880): 218. This anonymous New York pharmacist also pointed out that it was impossible to make a living without selling patent medicines.

14. Thousands of doctors were guilty of this, according to a report in the *New York Times*, 7 June 1882, p. 4, col. 7.

15. Samuel M. Colcord, "Professional Intercourse between the Apothecary and Physician," *Druggists Circular* 2 (1858): 58–59.

16. C. A. Lindsley, "The Prescription of Proprietary Medicines for the Sick—Its Demoralizing Effects on the Medical Profession," *Therapeutic Gazette* 6 (1882): 361–368.

17. "Neglect of the United States Pharmacopoeia," *Druggists Circular* 31 (1887): 208.

18. "Hap-Hazard Medications," *Druggists Circular* 31 (1887): 275.

19. Frank B. Hardesty, "Proprietary Medicines, Physicians and the Public from the Standpoint of a Pharmacist," *Druggists Circular* 50 (1906): 324–325.

20. "Secrets of the Druggists," *New York Times*, 11 June 1882, p. 10, cols. 4–5.

21. W. A. Puckner, "The Nostrum from the Viewpoint of the Pharmacist," *JAMA* 46 (1906): 1340–1341.

22. Miner L. H. Leavitt, "What Is the Duty of the Professional Pharmacist Regarding Patent Medicines?" *Druggists Circular* 35 (1891): 151–152; Harry M. Archer, "The Wholesale Prescribing of Manufactured Medicines," *Medical Record* 37 (1890): 164. Archer thought a large part of the problem was that many doctors were embarrassed by their ignorance of Latin and therefore used proprietaries to avoid revealing their deficiencies. "The Influence of Proprietary Pharmacy upon the Practice of Medicine," *Boston Medical and Surgical Journal* 120 (1889): 11–15.

23. David Cowen, "Pharmacists and Physicians: An Uneasy Relationship," *Pharmacy in History* 34 (1992): 3–16.

24. Otto Wall, "Manufacturers' Preparations Ordered in Prescriptions," *Proceedings of the American Pharmaceutical Association* 32 (1884): 428–431, 540. Wall was a doctor, pharmacist, and teacher and had a unique perspective on the situation.

25. "Substitution of Drugs in Prescriptions by Druggists," *Medical Record* 29 (1886): 15.

26. "Blunders in Drugs," *New York Tribune*, 17 July 1890, p. 6, col. 3.

27. C. Rufus Rorem and Robert P. Fischelis, *The Costs of Medicines* (Chicago: University of Chicago Press, 1932), 43.

28. "East River Medical Association," *Medical Record* 3 (1868–1869): 497–499; "The Renewal of Prescriptions," *Medical Record* 3 (1868–1869): 517–518. Also see John Ordronaux, "Physicians and Apothecaries, in Relation to the Repetition of Prescriptions without Authority," *Medical Record* 3 (1868–1869): 281–283; Ordronaux, "Renewal of Prescriptions," *Medical Record* 3 (1868–1869): 525–526; Frederic H. Gerrish, "The Ownership of Prescriptions," *Boston Medical and Surgical Journal* 103 (1880): 559–562.

29. *New York Times*, 29 April 1883, p. 8, cols. 6–7; *New York Times*, 24 August 1882, p. 4, col. 6.

30. Charles Greene, "The Relation of Druggist and Physician," *JAMA* 19 (1892): 719–721.

31. William C. Kirchgessner, "Developing a Prescription Business," *Proceedings of the American Pharmaceutical Association* 52 (1904): 207–213.

32. Sonnedecker, *History of Pharmacy* , 290.

33. William B. Lillard, "The Sale of Patent Medicines," *Druggists Circular* 31 (1887): 220. It seems he did not lose his job, however.

34. Sonnedecker, *History of Pharmacy*, 201–202.

35. How many of these were pharmacy graduates was not stated. "Number of Druggists in the United States by Decades," *Druggists Circular* 51 (1907): 155.

36. Advertisement in *Fayette Watch Tower*, August 1857.

37. Edward R. Squibb, "Prices of Dispensing Pharmacists," *Ephemeris* 2 (1885): 823–827. Squibb apparently did not count the owner's salary as part of the store's expenses, a common error according to a handbook published in 1913. D.

Charles O'Connor, *A Treatise on Commercial Pharmacy Intended as a Reference Book and a Textbook for Pharmacists and Their Clerks* (Philadelphia: Lippincott, 1913).

38. "Physic by the Wholesale," *Therapeutic Gazette* 6 (1882): 461–462.

39. A. W. Herzog, "Shall Physicians Dispense Their Own Medicines?" *New York Medical Journal* 53 (1891): 687–688.

40. "Family vs. Patent Medicines," *Pharmaceutical Era* 8 (1892): 4.

41. "Physicians vs. Pharmacists," *Druggists Circular* 30 (1886): 73.

42. "Don't Dose Yourself," *New York Tribune*, 11 October 1896, sect. 3, p. 1, cols. 5–6.

43. Daybooks of the Niagara Apothecary, Archives of the Province of Ontario, F1373 MS661, no. 3.

44. Some years later, in fact, the National Association of Retail Druggists (NARD) estimated that a headache remedy using acetphenetidin (Phenacetin) would cost eleven cents for one hundred powders; the total cost (packages, labels, other ingredients) for one dozen boxes of twenty-five-cent powders, packed one dozen to the box, was sixty-five cents. Otto Bruder, ed., *The Modern Pharmacist* (Chicago: NARD, 1910), 51. The cost of acetphenetidin at this time was about thirty-three cents per ounce.

45. The *Dental Register*, for example, seems to have confined its discussion of Antipyrine to an article on how the drug discolored the teeth: "Blackening of Teeth by Antipyrine," *Dental Register* 46 (1892): 262.

46. F. W. Haussmann, "Antikamnia," *American Journal of Pharmacy* 63 (1891): 181–182.

47. W. A. Hall, "An Examination of Antikamnia," *Druggists Circular* 35 (1891): 99.

48. Antikamnia Chemical Company, "Analyses of Antikamnia," *Druggists Circular* 35 (1891): 161.

49. See William C. Fiedler, "Antikamnia: The Story of a Pseudo-ethical Pharmaceutical," *Pharmacy in History* 21 (1979): 59–72.

50. For example, one of the headache powders most criticized by the muckrakers was a product named Orangeine, but it seems not to have been advertised in any well-known paper or magazine and was rarely advertised in any pharmaceutical periodical of which I am aware. Yet Edith Wharton mentioned it in *The House of Mirth* (1905), when a sweatshop seamstress recommended it to a colleague with a headache (book 2, chap. 10). It was still on the market as late as the 1970s, according to an undated document ("Internal Analgesics Products List") on file at the Consumer Health-Care Products Association (CHPA) offices in Washington, D.C.

51. See, for example, "Specialties for Counter Sale," *American Druggist* 36 (1900): 4. This article was in fact a prize essay, which suggests the importance of headache remedies for retail business.

52. "Dangers of Headache Powders, with Tests for Suspected Ingredients," *Therapeutic Gazette* 23 (1899): 758–759.

53. "Headache Powders in Western Pennsylvania," *Pharmaceutical Era* 22 (1899): 258.

54. David L. Edsall, "Headache," *Boston Medical and Surgical Journal* 174 (1916): 284–285. Doctors also sometimes prescribed a drug in quantity, and patients consequently took too much at one time. A headache prescription for bulk acetanilid, for example, resulted in one patient spending several days in a cyanotic state. G. Baringer Slifer, "A Case of Acetanilid Poisoning," *Therapeutic Gazette* 21 (1897): 360.

55. A. E. Austin and R. C. Larrabee, "Acetanilid Poisoning from the Use of Proprietary Headache Powders," *JAMA* 46 (1906): 1680–1681.

56. "Unethical Pharmaceutical Houses," *JAMA* 39 (1902): 1597; J. M. Anders, "The 'Patent Medicine' and Nostrum Evils," *JAMA* 46 (1906): 267–270.

57. "Relations of Pharmacy to the Medical Profession," *JAMA* 34 (1900): 986–988, 1049–1051, 1114–1116, 1178–79, 1327–1329, 1405–1407; 35 (1900): 27–29, 89–91. The editors initially promised to include an article on patented chemicals but it never appeared.

58. James Burrow, *AMA: Voice of American Medicine* (Baltimore: Johns Hopkins University Press, 1963), 71.

59. Ibid., 73; "Secret Nostrums and the Journal," *JAMA* 34 (1900): 1420.

60. Richard Hofstadter, *The Age of Reform: From Bryan to F.D.R.* (New York: Vintage Books, 1955), 185.

61. See C. C. Regier, *The Era of the Muckrakers* (Gloucester, Mass.: Peter Smith, 1957); Arthur Weinberg and Lila Weinberg, eds., *The Muckrakers* (New York: Simon and Schuster, 1961); Judson Grenier, "Muckraking and the Muckrakers: An Historical Definition," *Journalism Quarterly* 37 (1960): 552–558; Lewis Filler, *Crusaders for American Liberalism* (Yellow Springs, Ohio: Antioch Press, 1939).

62. The *Ladies' Home Journal*, however, usually discussed the items in general terms and only rarely identified an offending product or manufacturer by name.

63. Samuel Hopkins Adams, *The Great American Fraud: Articles on the Nostrum Evil and Quackery* (Chicago: American Medical Association, 1912), 3. The original article, titled "The Nostrum Evil," appeared in *Collier's,* 7 October 1905.

64. Ibid., 4, 34–35.

65. "How the Private Confidences of Women Are Laughed At," *Ladies' Home Journal,* November 1904, 18. Bok was in principle, of course, not opposed to advertising: only 30 out of 220 pages of his publication were entirely free of advertisements. John Drewry, *Some Magazines and Magazine Makers* (Boston: Strattford Co., 1924), 18–23.

66. See Salma Harja Steinberg, *Reformer in the Marketplace: Edward W. Bok and "The Ladies' Home Journal"* (Baton Rouge: Louisiana State University Press, 1979).

67. "Why Forty-five Women Died," *Ladies' Home Journal,* July 1906, 16. The most prominent physician who opposed all use of acetanilid was Abraham Jacobi, a well-known pediatrician. See A. Jacobi, "A Protest against Acetanilid," *JAMA* 46 (1906): 135.

68. "To You: A Personal Word," *Ladies' Home Journal*, February 1906, 20.

69. See, for example, J. R. Johns, "The Therapy of Acetanilid," *American Medicine* 7 (1904): 825–826. See also Richard Cabot, "The Physician's Responsibility for the Nostrum Evil," *JAMA* 47 (1906): 982–983. He said doctors "educated" their patients to take drugs when they really should be reforming their habits and lifestyles.

70. See, for example, Alfred Stengel, "Chronic Acetanilid Poisoning: Report of Two Additional Cases," *JAMA* 45 (1905): 243–245. One young man allegedly died after only one dose; "Danger in Headache Powders," *Druggists Circular* 50 (1906): 231. A young woman died after ingesting seven and a half grains; A. L. Smedley, "Death from Acetanilid Poisoning," *JAMA* 48 (1907): 1433. Lyman Kebler, "The Present Status of Drug Addiction in the United States," *Transactions of the American Therapeutic Society* 10 (1910): 105–119. Kebler looked at heroin as well as the antipyretic analgesics. From 1907 to 1923 he was head of the Bureau of Chemistry's drug division, which was charged with enforcing the new law. But see Martin Gross, *Acetanilid: A Critical Bibliographic Review* (New Haven, Conn.: Hillhouse Press, 1946), 58–103; Gross doubts the validity of any of these reports of deaths.

71. W. H. Graves, "Headache Powders and Deaths from Heart Disease," *JAMA* 46 (1906): 1221.

72. "Headache," *JAMA* 52 (1909): 1334–1335.

73. James Cassedy, "Muckraking and Medicine: Samuel Hopkins Adams," *American Quarterly* 16 (1964): 85–99.

74. "The Patent Medicine Men Active," *JAMA* 42 (1904): 1629.

75. "The Dangers of Self-Drugging," *JAMA* 44 (1905): 1041.

76. *American Medicine* 10 (1905): 1010.

77. W. H. Graves, "Teach the Public That Medical Practice Is More Than Drug-Giving," *JAMA* 48 (1907): 1617.

78. For a general overview, see Kenneth O. Peake, "Muckraking, Proprietary Medicine Advertising and the Pure Food and Drugs Act: A Study of Interrelationships," M.A. thesis, California State University, 1976.

79. William Rothstein, *American Physicians in the Nineteenth Century: From Sects to Science* (Baltimore: Johns Hopkins University Press, 1972), 317.

80. H. Wayne Morgan, *Drugs in America: A Social History, 1800–1980* (Syracuse: Syracuse University Press, 1981), 105.

81. James G. Burrow, "The Prescription-Drug Policies of the American Medical Association in the Progressive Era," in *Safeguarding the Public: Historical Aspects of Medicinal Drug Control*, ed. J. B. Blake (Baltimore: Johns Hopkins University Press, 1970).

82. John Ritter, "Pharmacopeial or Proprietary Prescriptions: Which?" *JAMA* 47

(1906): 683–684. See also M. I. Wilbert, The Elimination of the Nostrum Traffic, an Evident Duty of American Physicians," *JAMA* 46 (1906): 188–190.

83. J. H. Long, "Why the Work of the Council on Pharmacy and Chemistry Is Necessary," *JAMA* 46 (1906): 1344–1345; Burrow, *AMA*, 74–75. Also see Joseph C. Aub and Ruth K. Hapgood, *Pioneer in Modern Medicine: David Linn Edsall of Harvard* (Cambridge: Harvard Medical Alumni Association, 1970), 42ff., which discusses the formation of the council.

84. See *JAMA* 44 (1905): 720–721. The rules also appear in the *New York Medical Journal* 81 (1905): 452.

85. The law was summarized by J. H. Beal, "A Synopsis, with Comments, of the Principal Provisions of the Federal Pure Food and Drug Law," *Proceedings of the American Pharmaceutical Association* 54 (1906): 202–215. Also see Oscar E. Anderson, Jr., *The Health of a Nation: Harvey W. Wiley and the Fight for Pure Food* (Chicago: University of Chicago Press for University of Cincinnati Press, 1958); Harry Edward Neal, *The Protectors: The Story of the Food and Drug Administration* (New York: Julian Messner, 1968); Peter Temin, *Taking Your Medicine: Drug Regulation in the United States* (Cambridge: Harvard University Press, 1980); Robert Valuck, Suzanne Poirier, and Robert Mrtek, "Patent Medicine Muckraking: Influences on American Pharmacy, Social Reform, and Foreign Authors," *Pharmacy in History* 34 (1992): 183–192; Mitchell Okun, *Fair Play in the Marketplace: The First Battle for Pure Food and Drugs* (De Kalb: Northern Illinois University Press, 1986); Lorine S. Goodwin, *The Pure Food, Drink, and Drug Crusaders, 1879–1914* (Jefferson, N.C.: McFarland, 1999); James Harvey Young, "Federal Drug and Narcotic Regulation," *Pharmacy in History* 37 (1995): 59–67.

86. See Paul Starr, *The Social Transformation of American Medicine: The Rise of a Sovereign Profession and the Making of a Vast Industry* (New York: Basic Books, 1982), 127ff.; David Dykstra, "The Medical Profession and Patent and Proprietary Medicines during the Nineteenth Century," *Bulletin of the History of Medicine* 29 (1955): 401–419. Contemporaries also praised the AMA's participation in this event; J. H. Carstens, "The Future of the Medical Profession," *Cincinnati Lancet-Clinic* 96 (1906): 521–525.

87. See James Harvey Young, *The Medical Messiahs: A Social History of Health Quackery in Twentieth-Century America* (Princeton: Princeton University Press, 1967), chap. 1, in which he discusses the immediate impact of the 1906 act.

88. "History of the Proprietary Association from 1881," uncataloged compilation, CHPA, Washington, D.C.

89. PAA, Executive Committee Minutes, 7 October 1907, CHPA, Washington, D.C. At least one member resigned, however, because the PAA did not go far enough in complying with the spirit of the new law; letter from Charles H. Stowell, treasurer and general manager of J. C. Ayers Company, *Druggists Circular* 50 (1906): 101. The PAA was quite righteous in its defense of its own good intentions, but the organization represented only a fraction of the nostrum companies in the

United States, and its members might be said to be of the better class of manufacturers.

90. Concerned individuals who thought the synthetics were safe also published pamphlets saying so, but it is impossible to tell if a manufacturer was ultimately behind them. See, for example, Uriel Boone, *Antipyrine, Acetanilide and Phenacetin: Are They Harmful Remedies? Are They Habit-Forming Drugs?* (privately published, after 1909). Boone (who does not identify himself further) had conducted a survey of the use of these drugs in hospitals and found them to be without danger.

91. PAA, Executive Committee Minutes, 7 September 1916, CHPA, Washington, D.C.

92. The 1905 census indicates this was the total value of proprietaries. "Government Statistics concerning Manufacturing Druggists," *Druggists Circular* 51 (1907): 154–155. "Druggists' preparations" (loosely defined as prescription pharmaceuticals) were valued at $31.8 million—less than half the value of patent medicines.

93. Frank J. Cheney, "The Proprietary Medicine Industry," *Pharmaceutical Era* 45 (1912): 637–640. The PAA also apparently resolved in 1915 to remove "cures" from its members' advertising and to stop selling anything as an abortifacient. But in the 1920s the association represented less than 10 percent of the country's nostrum manufacturers, although this was 60 percent of the companies making the most money. Ervin Kemp, "Some Notes on the History of the Proprietary Association," *Journal of the American Pharmaceutical Association* 15 (1926): 973–979.

94. "Physicians and the Food and Drugs Act," *JAMA* 48 (1907): 241–24; Carstens, "Future of the Medical Profession"; William J. Mayo, "The Medical Profession and the Issues Which Confront It," *Boston Medical and Surgical Journal* 154 (1906): 667–671.

95. There is a fairly extensive literature on drug addiction and the part narcotics have played in American life. Among the best are Morgan, *Drugs in America*; David F. Musto, *The American Disease: Origins of Narcotics Control*, 2nd ed. (New York: Oxford University Press, 1987); David Courtwright, *Dark Paradise: Opiate Addiction in America before 1940* (Cambridge: Harvard University Press, 1982). For contemporary views, consult Edward Levinstein, *Morbid Craving for Morphia*, trans. C. Harrer (1878; reprint, New York: Arno Press, 1981); H. H. Kane, *Drugs That Enslave: The Opium, Morphine, Chloral, and Hashisch Habits* (Philadelphia: Presley Blakiston, 1881). On the 1914 law, see also Edward M. Brecher, *Licit and Illicit Drugs* (Boston: Little, Brown, 1972), 48–55. Small quantities of opiates in over-the-counter medications were still permitted until 1970.

96. See Starr, *Social Transformation*, 116–123, in which he discusses the Flexner report, the survey of medical schools that revealed the abysmal conditions in many of them. The best schools were almost always regular, and the report was a great boost to the AMA and other reformers; Abraham Flexner, *Medical Education in the United States and Canada* (New York: Carnegie Foundation for

Advancement of Teaching, 1910). J. H. Salisbury, "The Subordination of Medical Journals to Proprietary Interests," *JAMA* 46 (1906): 1337–1338; George H. Simmons, "The Commercial Domination of Therapeutics and the Movement for Reform," *JAMA* 48 (1907): 1645–1653.

97. *American Medicine* 10 (1905): 1.

98. "Council on Pharmacy and Chemistry, American Medical Association," *Boston Medical and Surgical Journal* 152 (1905): 288–289.

99. "The Possible Failure of the American Medical Association's Inquisition Concerning Proprietaries," *New York Medical Journal* 81 (1905): 656.

100. Francis Pottenger, "Some Observations on the Present Status of American Medical Journalism," *Transactions of the American Therapeutic Society* 15 (1915): 19–24.

101. R. O. Semmes, "The Medical Profession and the Medical Journals in Relation to Nostrums," *Boston Medical and Surgical Journal* 15 (1906): 331. Semmes was the county health officer for Wilcox, Alabama.

102. "The Work of the Manufacturing Druggist," *New York Medical Journal* 88 (1908): 848.

103. "Another Phase of the Proprietary Question," *Massachusetts Medical Journal* 26 (1906): 382. This editorial was taken from another journal. The CPC had pronounced both Anasarcin and Antiphlogistine to be unethical.

104. Graham Hereford, "Combines Efficacy with Safety," *Massachusetts Medical Journal* 26 (1906): 365.

105. "The Conspiracy of Silence," *JAMA* 58 (1912): 36–37.

106. See Fiedler, "Antikamnia"; "Acetphenetidin Labeling Decision," *Journal of Industrial and Engineering Chemistry* 3 (1911): 528.

107. Edgar Allen Forbes, "What Not to Do for a Headache," *World's Work* 20 (1910): 13081–13083.

108. *Druggists Circular* 51 (1907): 292.

109. "To Fight Headache Powders," *Pharmaceutical Era* 45 (1912): 204; "Lays Heart Disease to Coal-Tar 'Cures,'" *New York Times*, 26 March 1910, p. 2, col. 6.

110. "How the Sale of Headache Remedies Is Pushed," *JAMA* 49 (1907): 1381–1382.

111. A. Emil Hiss and Albert E. Ebert, *The New Standard Formulary* (Chicago: Engelhard, 1912), 577–578.

112. "'Headache Cures' and the Druggist," *Druggists Circular* 55 (1911): 67.

113. On the topic of price-cutting, see George Seabury, *Shall Pharmacists Become Tradesmen?* (New York: George Seabury, 1899). Seabury thought price-cutting was a major impediment to professional practice and devoted most of his book to a discussion of the subject.

An earlier version of NARD had been short-lived. George Urdang, "The Precedents of the N.A.R.D. and Its Founding Fifty Years Ago," *American Journal of Pharmaceutical Education*, April 1949.

114. Valuck, Poirier, and Mrtek, "Patent Medicine Muckraking."

115. "Mr. Bok Again," *Bulletin of Pharmacy* 19 (1905): 271; "Mr. Bok and His Troubles," 444; "Reforms Likely to Result," 445.

116. Henry Strong, *The Machinations of the American Medical Association: An Exposure and a Warning* (St. Louis: National Druggist, 1909), 34. In the original the entire passage is in boldface. Strong's *National Druggist* was financed by the PAA. David Cowen and William Helfand, "The Progressive Movement and Its Impact on Pharmacy," *Pharmaceutica Acta Helvetica* 54 (1979): 317–323.

117. See *Pharmaceutical Era* 22 (1899): 20. "Safe Headache Remedy," *Druggists Circular* 57 (1913): 459.

118. Otto Bruder, ed., *The Modern Pharmacist* (Chicago: NARD, 1910), 121–122.

119. His store also sold about a hundred thousand tablets containing one or the other of the coal tar products to the one hundred doctors with whom he did business. F. M. Higgins, "The Druggists' Duty Concerning Coal-Tar," *Druggists Circular* 56 (1912): 512–513.

120. Unfortunately for this point of view, headache remedies were also part of the grocery store business in some states. The *Druggists Circular* found this intolerable: "Just why a grocery store should be allowed to sell 'headache powders,' whether pure or impure, is a matter which might properly form the subject of an inquiry by the board of pharmacy or the board of health"; "Dangers in Headache Powders," *Druggists Circular* 50 (1906): 231. See also "The Pharmacopeial Grocer," *Druggists Circular* 36 (1892): 260. Pharmacists, unlike grocers, were *legally* responsible for the quality of the goods they sold and were trained to detect adulterants and impurities. Allowing drugs to be sold alongside bread and canned tomatoes might suggest to the public that the medicines were as innocuous as the food. In fact, in the 1930s, the same journal was expressing the same annoyance about the same issues. Lounsbury Pyne, "Drugs in Grocery Stores," *Druggists Circular* 77 (1933): 14–15, 58–60.

121. For a discussion of the perspective that industrial production was contributing to pharmaceutical autonomy, see J. K. Crellin, "Industrial Pharmacy: A Divisive Force between Medicine and Pharmacy in the Early Twentieth Century?" in *Farmacía e industralizacion*, ed. F.J.P. Sarmiento (Madrid: Sociedad Española de Historia de la Farmacía, 1985).

CHAPTER 6   THE BAYER COMPANY

1. Kurt Witthauer, "Aspirin, ein neues Salicylpräparat," *Therapeutische Monatsheft* 13 (1899): 330; Julius Wohlgemuth, "Über Aspirin (Acetylsalicylsäure)," *Therapeutische Monatsheft* 13 (1899): 276–279; Heinrich Dreser, "Pharmakologisches über Aspirin (Acetylsalicylsäure)," *Pflügers Archiv* 76 (1899): 306–318.

2. Alfred Hauser, "Geschichte der Verkaufsabteilung Pharma Bayer," 4ff., 1/6.6.18, Bayer Archiv Leverkusen (BAL).

3. "Zum Wortschutz 'Phenacetin,'" *Pharmazeutische Zeitung* 41 (1896): 307;

"Nochmals zum Wortschutz 'Phenacetin,'" *Pharmazeutische Zeitung* 41 (1896): 609.

4. Bayer had been involved in American chemical manufacturing since 1871 and bought a plant in Rensselaer, New York, in 1903, which began to produce drug chemicals soon thereafter. The only full-scale study of Bayer in America is Thomas M. Reimer, "Bayer and Company in the United States: German Dyes, Drugs and Cartels in the Progressive Era," Ph.D. dissertation, Syracuse University, 1996. This work has been most useful in helping sort out the complex history of this firm. See also Williams Haynes, *The American Chemical Industry*, 6 vols. (New York: Van Nostrand, 1945–1954), 1:308, 6:174–175; E. Hendrick, "Record of the Coal-Tar Color Industry at Albany," *Journal of Industrial and Engineering Chemistry* 16 (1924): 411–413.

5. See Reimer, "Bayer," chap. 4.

6. William Henry Becker, "The Wholesalers of Hardware and Drugs, 1870–1900," Ph.D. dissertation, Johns Hopkins University, 1969, 221. At midcentury, *Nelson's Northern Lancet* (2 [1852]: 80) had recommended Schieffelin in an editorial, and the advertisement in that issue indicated the company had its own laboratory to ensure scientific production of pure products.

7. E. N. Gathercoal, *The Prescription Ingredient Survey* (Chicago: APhA, 1933), 8. An analysis of twelve thousand prescriptions in 1895 in fact indicated that Phenacetin was the most prescribed proprietary product in the country.

8. Charles C. Mann and Mark L. Plummer, *The Aspirin Wars: Money, Medicine, and One Hundred Years of Rampant Competition* (New York: Alfred A. Knopf, 1991), 29. See Reimer, "Bayer," 52ff. Reimer also provides the details of Bayer's business arrangements as it developed its American operation.

9. H. Schweitzer to I.J.R. Muurling, 4 February 1897, Alien Property Custodian (APC), RG 131, entry 199, case 4062, box 162, National Archives, Washington, D.C. Bayer's U.S. patents were held by its counsel, E. N. Dickerson.

10. Reimer, "Bayer," 131, quoting the *Boettingerchronik*, an in-house history of Bayer written in 1909.

11. "Schieffelin and Co. No Longer Agents for Products of Farbenfabriken of Elberfeld," *Pharmaceutical Era* 19 (1898): 915.

12. Although other German companies also charged prices that annoyed the pharmacists, Bayer was the one firm that was always singled out (by product, if not by company name) for the most scathing comments. See J. Pfeiffer, "What Legislation Can Be Proposed to Check the Exorbitant Charges Made in This Country, by Foreign Manufacturers, on the So-called Patented Chemicals, as Compared with Prices Asked in Other Countries?" *Pharmaceutical Era* 21 (1899): 758.

13. "Phenacetin at Auction," *New York Tribune*, 16 December 1897, p. 2, col. 4.

14. "The Phenacetine Litigations," *Pharmaceutical Era* 19 (1898): 4–5.

15. "Phenacetine Smuggler on Trial," *Pharmaceutical Era* 19 (1898): 405; "More Drug Smuggling Cases," *Pharmaceutical Era* 19 (1898): 597.

16. "Phenacetine Smuggling," *Windsor Evening Record*, 29 December 1898, p. 1, col. 2.

17. "How It Is Done," *Pharmaceutical Era* 19 (1898): 696. Canadian pharmacists were notified in 1898 "that in future phenacetine must not be accepted for entry into [the United States] except that brought in by the authorized selling agents. This is a move of some importance to Canadian dealers, as heretofore considerable quantities had been shipped from here. The only result will be a great increase of smuggling, as the temptation to do so on account of the difference in price is very great"; *Canadian Pharmaceutical Journal* 32 (1898): 13.

18. "Valuable Drugs Seized in a Room on Howard Street," *Detroit Journal*, 15 February 1900, clipping, file C38 (a)I, Farbenfabriken of Elberfeld Co., Kremers Reference Files (KRF), University of Wisconsin, Madison.

19. A. C. Smith communicated his thoughts in a letter to the *Pharmaceutical Review*, 29 May 1905; found in file C38 (a)I, Farbenfabriken of Elberfeld Co., KRF. His letterhead, at least, called him an "Importer of Fine Chemicals." But more on Mr. Smith later in the chapter.

20. "Enjoined by United States Court," *Cincinnati Enquirer*, 8 December 1899, clipping, file C38 (a)I, Farbenfabriken of Elberfeld Co., KRF; there is also a clipping from the *Macon News*, 19 May 1903, titled "Phenacetine Agents Scour State to Bring Suit."

21. "Smuggling Phenacetine," *Pharmaceutical Era* 21 (1899): 18. George McMillan worked at Parke-Davis's Canadian location but roomed in Detroit. He was carrying five hundred ounces.

22. "Heavily Punished for Selling Phenacetin in Violation of An Injunction," *Pharmaceutical Era* 21 (1899): 92.

23. "More Phenacetine Cases East and West," *Pharmaceutical Era* 19 (1898): 797.

24. Reimer, "Bayer," 131.

25. *Pharmaceutical Era* 19 (1898).

26. Reimer tells the rather convoluted story of the law suits, appeals, injunctions, and reactions ("Bayer," 130–142).

27. Quotation cited from 108 *Federal Reporter* 233; upheld on appeal in February 1902, 113 *Federal Reporter* 870. See also Reimer, "Bayer," 133.

28. "A Decision in the Maurer Phenacetine Case," *Pharmaceutical Era* 26 (1901): 524.

29. "Phenacetine Suit Settled," *Pharmaceutical Era* 26 (1901): 697–698.

30. Reimer, "Bayer," 134.

31. Letter to the trade from Farbenfabriken of Elberfeld, 5 May 1900, file C38 (a)I, Farbenfabriken of Elberfeld Co., KRF. Bayer, in fact, sent most of the newspaper clippings that are now in the Kremers Reference Files to Edward Kremers in his capacity as editor of the *Pharmaceutical Review*. Presumably other respectable

journals were also contacted with similar requests and evidence of the serious-
ness with which Bayer treated smuggling cases.

32. Clipping from *Boston Traveler*, 3 December 1903, file C38 (a)I, Farbenfabriken of
Elberfeld Co., KRF.

33. Reimer, "Bayer," 137–140. See also "A Sensation," *Bulletin of Pharmacy* 17 (1903):
50–51: "Nothing has apparently been done to prosecute the alleged substitu-
tors, and it looks as though the newspaper exposition and publicity was the only
end held in view." See also "The Phenacetine Crusade," *Bulletin of Pharmacy* 17
(1903): 93. "The Moral," *Bulletin of Pharmacy* 17 (1903): 94, reminded druggists
that now the pharmacist "would be called upon to vouch for the purity and
quality of the drugs he compounds and dispenses, regardless of whom they may
be purchased."

34. Reimer, "Bayer," 143; "A. C. Smith's Record," *N.A.R.D. Notes* 38 (1 July 1905): 7–11;
"*Notes* Nails More of A. C. Smith's Lies," *N.A.R.D. Notes* 39 (8 July 1905): 7–11; "A.
C. Smith's 'Aristol' Frauds," *N.A.R.D. Notes* 40 (15 July 1905): 9–13.

35. Reimer, "Bayer," 141. For material on Monsanto and Mallinckrodt, see Dan J.
Forrestal, *Faith, Hope and $5,000: The Story of Monsanto; The Trials and Triumphs
of the First Seventy-five Years* (New York: Simon and Schuster, 1977), 21–23;
Haynes, *American Chemical Industry*, vol. 1, chap. 20; vol. 3, chap. 19. The American organic chemical industry was not significant so long as the German firms
were dominant, but as patents expired and as the possibility of a war in Europe
loomed, several U.S. chemical manufacturers (some of them already in the
drug trade) began to take an interest in local production. Haynes's work,
although dated and biased, is still a good source, especially volume 6, the company histories.

36. Gathercoal, *Prescription Ingredient Survey*, 26.

37. Prescription books, file C39q, KRF.

38. This pharmacist had deliberately dispensed generic acetphenetidin instead of
Phenacetin because in his professional opinion the drugs were chemically identical. For his trouble, he received a visit from the representatives of "a large German chemical house," who told him he had broken the law. This visit, of course,
had more to do with issues related to smuggling and counterfeiting, but he was
angry at the "remarkable powers" the patent laws had given manufacturers.
William C. Alpers, "Substitution and the Mann Bill," *Druggists Circular* 49 (1905):
110–111.

39. This volume was scheduled to appear in 1900 but was delayed until 1905.

40. Adolf G. Vogeler, "Patented Synthetics in the *Pharmacopoeia*," *Western Druggist* 21
(1899): 483, quoting the AMA's resolution. The AMA seems to have neglected to
report on this meeting in its own journal. There is only the briefest mention of
its having taken place.

41. Charles Rice, "The Recognition of Synthetics and Introduction of Doses," *Ameri-

can Druggist 36 (1900): 261–263. See also Adolf G. Vogeler, "Patented Synthetics in the *Pharmacopoeia*," *Western Druggist* 21 (1899): 483–484.

42. M92-347, Committee of Revision Circular 334, 16 February 1900, "General Principles of Upcoming Revision," United States Pharmacopeial Convention (USPC) Collection, State Historical Society of Wisconsin Archives, Madison.

43   M92-347, Committee of Revision Circular 335, n.d., "Remarks on the Provisional Draft of the 'General Principles' Proposed in Circular 334," USPC Collection.

44. M92-347, Committee of Revision Circular 503, 4 April 1904, USPC Collection.

45. M92-347, Committee of Revision Circular 518, 25 July 1904, USPC Collection.

46. M92-347, Committee of Revision Circular 514, 22 July 1904, and Committee of Revision Circular 524, 29 July 1904, both in USPC Collection.

47. *The Pharmacopoeia of the United States of America*, 8th rev. ed. (Philadelphia: P. Blakiston's, 1905), 428–429.

48. M92-347, Committee of Revision Circular 573, 23 September 1904, USPC Collection.

49. John M. Francis, "The New *Pharmacopoeia*," *Bulletin of Pharmacy* 19 (1906): 273–276 and passim; S. W. Williams, "Impressions of the New *Pharmacopoeia*," *Druggists Circular* 49 (1905): 307–309; F. J. Wulling, "The 1900 *Pharmacopoeia*," *Northwestern Druggist* 6 (1905): 17–20; "The Purgation of Therapeutics," *Boston Medical and Surgical Journal* 154 (1906): 252–253.

50. "*Pharmacopoeia* Condemned," *Medical News* 87 (1905): 1276. J. Leverett of Yonkers agreed: "The *Pharmacopoeia*—As Seen by One General Practitioner," *Massachusetts Medical Journal* 27 (1907): 310–311.

51. "Trade Names in the New *Pharmacopoeia*," *Druggists Circular* 49 (1905): 301–303. Others might not have seen a conspiracy but did note "the rather indifferent way in which many of the clear and definite instructions to the Committee of Revision have been carried out" with respect to the synthetics. M. I. Wilbert, "A Review of the Eighth Decennial Revision of the Pharmacopoeia of the United States of America," *American Journal of Pharmacy* 77 (1905): 356.

52. H. G. Posey, "The Official Names for Controlled Synthetics," *Druggists Circular* 49 (1905): 400. This druggist was in fact "red-headed" about what Bayer had done to keep its trade names.

53. See J. R. Remington, "Prescription Difficulties," *American Druggist* 52 (1908): 33–34; George Simmons, "The Commercial Domination of Therapeutics and the Movement for Reform," *JAMA* 48 (1907): 1645–1653.

54. "Wie beschützen wir unsere Produkte nach Ablauf der Patente?" undated typescript, APC, RG 131, entry 199, case file 4062, box 162, p. 5, National Archives.

55. Ibid. Although the Antikamnia Company began to substitute phenacetin for acetanilid as a consequence of the Food and Drug Act, this was not the company identified by Bayer. The Antikamnia Company purchased its acetphenetidin from Monsanto. As we saw in chapter 5, Antikamnia went to court over

phenacetin labeling, in 1914 losing once and for all the right not to list it. Also see Reimer, "Bayer," 124.

56. In 1926 there were 384.8 orders for acetphenetidin (including 271.4 for phenacetin) per 10,000 prescriptions, an increase from 227.4 in 1909 (all of which were for phenacetin) (Gathercoal, *Prescription Ingredient Survey*, 29).

57. The overproduction of acetanilid in anticipation of a need that did not materialize led to a price war, but despite some losses, Bayer's sales of phenacetin after 1906 remained healthy. Quality was still important, and Bayer had never lost its reputation for high-caliber products. Reimer, "Bayer," 125.

58. "Phenacetin, Sulphonal and Trional," *JAMA* 58 (1912): 1298–1299.

59. Martin Gross and Leon Greenberg, *The Salicylates: A Critical Bibliographic Review* (New Haven, Conn.: Hillhouse Press, 1948); Bayer AG, *Aspirin, ein Jahrhundert-pharmakon: Daten, Fakten, Perspektiven* (Leverkusen: Bayer, 1983), 24ff.; Arthur Eichengrün, "Pharmazeutisch-wissenschaftliche Abteilung," in "Geschichte und Entwicklung der Farbenfabriken vorm: Friedr. Bayer & Co. Elberfeld in den ersten 50 Jahren (1863–1913)," manuscript, Leverkusen, 1918, 409ff.; Arthur Eichengrün, "50 Jahre Aspirin," *Pharmazie* 4 (1949): 582–584. Eichengrün's second article gives a very different picture from the first one. See also J. McTavish, "The German Pharmaceutical Industry, 1880–1920: A Case Study of Aspirin," M.A. thesis, University of Minnesota, 1986, 60–63; Mann and Plummer, *Aspirin Wars*, 25–28; Kim D. Rainsford, *Aspirin and the Salicylates* (London: Butterworth's, 1984); John R. Vane and Regina M. Botting, eds., *Aspirin and Other Salicylates* (London: Chapman and Hall Medical, 1992).

60. *American Journal of Pharmacy* 74 (1902): 442–443.

61. For example, James Burnet found Aspirin to be effective in alleviating certain kinds of cancer pain: "The Therapeutics of Aspirin and Mesotan," *Lancet* 1 (1905): 1193–1196. See also F. Merkel, "Aspirin als Analgeticum in der Gynäkologie und Geburtshilfe," *Deutsches Archiv für Klinische Medizin* 84 (1905): 261–264; R. T. Williamson, "On the Treatment of Glycosuria and Diabetes mellitus with Aspirin," *British Medical Journal* 2 (1902): 1946–1948. The first American use of Aspirin was reported by F. G. Floeckinger of Texas: "An Experimental Study of Aspirin, a New Salicylic Acid Preparation," *Medical News* 75 (1899): 645–647. See also Gross and Greenberg, *Salicylates*. They list just over four thousand titles that had appeared on this topic since antiquity. Many of them, of course, were responses to the discoveries of the late nineteenth century; a number of them deal with pre-ASA salicylates, but most discuss Aspirin. We discuss Aspirin's role in non-rheumatic headaches in the next chapter.

62. *Farbenfabriken v. Edward A. Kuehmsted*, APC, RG 131, entry 274 (Aspirin patent suits file), box 1, National Archives.

63. "*Farbenfabriken vormals Friedrich Bayer & Co. v. Chemische Fabrik von Heyden,*" *Reports of Patent, Design and Trade Mark Cases* 22 (1905): 501–518.

64. Seized records of the Farbenfabriken Co. regarding patent interference suits

brought in U.S. Courts, 1898–1913, APC, RG 131, entry 274, seized by the Alien Property Custodian (WWI) , National Archives.

65. "Aspirin—Acetylsalicylic Acid Patent Upheld," *Druggists Circular* 53 (1909): 496.

66. Unsigned memo on "Propaganda," 23 August 1911, from New York to Germany, APC, RG 131, entry 199, case 4062, box 162, National Archives. The company had in fact withdrawn its advertising (for all products) between 1 June and 1 October 1910.

67. Carl Duisberg and Rudolph Mann to Farbenfabriken of Elberfeld, 16 September 1911, APC, RG 131, entry 199, case file 4062, box 162, National Archives. In April 1907, Aspirin sales were around $11,800; by April 1910, they had jumped to about $25,200; and by September 1910, they amounted to about $38,300 out of a total of $70,700 spent on all pharmaceutical products that month, making Aspirin responsible for 54 percent of all pharmaceutical sales. Minutes of pharmaceutical conference, 4 October 1910, IV/80/III, BAL.

68. Lee Anderson and Gregory Higby summarize the discussions in *The Spirit of Voluntarism: A Legacy of Commitment and Contribution* (Rockville, Md.: USPC, 1995), 224ff. Among the other important items being considered were Hoechst's Novocaine (procaine) and Parke-Davis's Adrenalin (epinephrine).

69. Subcommittee vote: letter 59, p. 22, 31 May 1911; executive committee votes: letter 79, p. 494, 22 July 1911; letter 194, p. 1068, 1 June 1912; MS 149, box 67, USPC Collection.

70. George H. Simmons to Joseph P. Remington, 20 July 1912, MS 149, box 17, folder 6, Correspondence, USPC Collection. ASA as a useful abbreviation was not proposed and does not seem to have been used until the 1920s, when it begins to appear in Canadian pharmaceutical advertising.

71. Joseph P. Remington to George H. Simmons, 23 July 1912, MS 149, box 17, folder 6, Correspondence, USPC Collection.

72. See Oliver T. Osborne, "A Last Plea for a Useful *Pharmacopoeia*," *JAMA* 60 (1913): 1427–1430; Osborne, "The Absurdities and the Commercialism of the Proposed Ninth Decennial Revision of the *United States Pharmacopoeia*," *JAMA* 60 (1913): 2039–2042. Osborne, a professor of therapeutics at Yale, was angry that the new *USP* would accept all sorts of useless items but omit things like Aspirin and Novocaine. He also suspected that the more drugs the book contained, the more money this meant for someone and that commercial interests were behind it.

73. Letter from Joseph P. Remington, letter 449, p. 2723, 2 May 1914, MS 149, box 69, folder 1, Letters of the Executive Committee of Revision, USPC Collection. Also see Anderson and Higby, *Spirit of Voluntarism*, 227.

74. Benjamin Solis-Cohen, note appended to letter of Joseph P. Remington, letter 511, p. 3001, 8 August 1914, MS 149, box 69, folder 2, USPC Collection.

75. Reimer, "Bayer," 143.

76. "Pharmaceutical Era Defends Integrity of Druggists," *Pharmaceutical Era* 45 (1912): 554–555; "Held for Selling Counterfeit 'Aspirin,'" *Pharmaceutical Era* 45 (1912): 602.

77. "Chemical Importers after the Druggists," *Druggists Circular* 56 (1912): 585.

78. "Metz Charges Wholesale Drug Frauds," *Pharmaceutical Era* 45 (1912): 602.

79. The substitution and smuggling problem is revealed in a report made by one of Bayer's employees, Dr. Segin, after his travels in the South. "Reisebericht Dr. Segin," undated, unsigned typescript [1913], APC, RG 131, entry 199, case file 4062, box 162, National Archives. See also A. A. Ransom, "Acetylsalicylic Acid and Aspirin," *JAMA* 59 (1912): 1642; Edgar L. Patch, "Report of the Committee on Drug Market," *Journal of the American Pharmaceutical Association* 2 (1913): 1081–1108.

80. There is also a photograph of the barn (complete with horse), and a good deal of red ink, as well as a reference to A. C. Smith, *Warning against the Criminal Traffic in Drugs by Peddlers* (New York: National Health Conservation League, ca. 1913), in file C39 (n), Adulteration and Counterfeiting, KRF.

81. Quoted in Reimer, "Bayer," 144.

82. Ibid. Even so, not all aspirin was Aspirin. In February 1914, Bayer sampled sixty purchases of Aspirin from Brooklyn, Chicago, Boston, Cleveland, and a few other cities but was happy to report that "only" sixteen of them "contained the infringing product." Minutes of pharmaceutical conference, 26 February 1914, II/80/XIII, BAL.

83. Minutes of pharmaceutical conference, 19 April 1910, p. 1, IV/80/III, BAL.

84. So said Dr. Segin, "Reisebericht": "'Farbenfabriken of Elberfeld Co.' ist für das amerikanische Idiom zungenbrecherisch und kaum zu halten."

85. Mann and Plummer, *Aspirin Wars*, 45–46. The creation of these two companies also had much to do with the fact that Farbenfabriken was being sued by American dye interests under antitrust legislation.

86. The *Canadian Druggist* listed Aspirin in 1913 at fifty cents per ounce; in the United States in 1914 it was still forty-three cents, according to the *Druggists Circular.*

87. For example, in 1909 the company sold 402,521 ounces of Aspirin directly to the retail trade (as a powder) and 283,952 ounces to tablet manufacturers. As of August the following year, 377,404 ounces had been sold to retailers and 347,696 ounces to other drug companies. Minutes of pharmaceutical conference, 4 October 1910, IV/80/III, BAL.

88. "Wie beschützen," 7–8. In the presence of iron chloride, free salicylic acid (considered to be the cause of stomach irritation) produced a violet-colored reaction, which might suggest that aspirin was actually salicylic acid and therefore not novel enough for a patent. In Germany, on the other hand, tablet technology worked in Bayer's favor because its competitors' tablets were often indigestible, exiting the body intact, like little stones. Jan R. McTavish, "Aspirin in Germany: The Pharmaceutical Industry and the Pharmaceutical Profession," *Pharmacy in History* 29 (1987): 103–115.

89. Minutes of pharmaceutical conference, 4 October 1910, IV/80/III, BAL.

90. For example, the Sears, Roebuck and Co. spring catalog for 1912 (p. 480) advertised a bottle of fifty-five-grain aspirin tablets for forty-two cents, but the entry does not include the name Bayer anywhere.

CHAPTER 7   DID THE HEADACHE FINALLY MEET ITS MATCH?

1. *New York Times*, 10 and 11 July 1916; *New York Tribune*, 10 July 1916.

2. *New York World*, 17 August 1916, 1ff.; 19 August, p. 2, cols. 3–4. Heyden had a factory in Garfield, N.J., established in 1900.

3. See Charles Mann and Mark L. Plummer, *The Aspirin Wars: Money, Medicine, and One Hundred Years of Rampant Competition* (New York: Alfred A. Knopf, 1991), 40–42. Also see John P. Jones and Paul M. Hollister, *The German Secret Service in America, 1914–1918* (Boston: Small Maynard, 1918), 214.

4. Thomas M. Reimer, "Bayer and Company in the United States: German Dyes, Drugs and Cartels in the Progressive Era," Ph.D. dissertation, Syracuse University, 1996, 196–236.

5. "Protokoll über die am Samstag, den 22. August 1914, abgehaltene Konferenz betreffend unseren Verkehr mit Amerika während des Krieges," 9/A.1, Bayer Archiv Leverkusen (BAL).

6. "Aspirin Held Not to Be a Trade-Mark," *Druggists Circular* 63 (1919): 36.

7. According to the July 1916 issue of the *Pharmaceutical Era*, the tablets appeared "in the early part of this year." "Patents on Aspirin Expire in 1917," *Pharmaceutical Era* 49 (1916): 227–228. Mann and Plummer (*Aspirin Wars*, 37) say that Bayer produced its tablets in early 1914, but the intracompany debate over tablets did not take place until August of that year, after the war in Europe had begun. Schweitzer's purchase of Edison's phenol, however, allowed Bayer to resume large-scale Aspirin production in late 1915.

8. Memorandum, undated (probably ca. 1910–1911), headed "The following propaganda methods originated with us: . . . 'Bayer-Bayer' Cross This was designed in 1902, and was afterwards adopted by Elberfeld and is now extensively used by them. It is considered of great importance in propaganda as a means of identification for the Bayer products," Alien Property Custodian (APC), RG 131, entry 199, case file 4062, box 162, National Archives, Washington, D.C.

9. See the story of "Fellow's Hypophosphites" told by George H. Simmons, "The Commercial Domination of Therapeutics," *JAMA* 48 (1907): 1645–1653. This had been an ordinary public nostrum with unremarkable sales until its owners then made it "ethical" and profits soared.

10. Vincent Vinikas, *Soft Soap, Hard Sell: American Hygiene in an Age of Advertisement* (Ames: Iowa State University Press, 1992), chap. 2.

11. "Edward Germann's Death," *New York Times*, 22 January 1906, p. 5. col. 6; "Veronal and Its Uses," 23 January 1906, p. 8, col. 4.

12. See "Wie beschützen wir unsere Produkte nach Ablauf der Patente?" typescript

(undated), APC, RG 131, entry 199, case file 4062, box 162, National Archives. Schweitzer had expressed much the same concerns in the spring of 1913 and considered the AMA a force to be reckoned with, but one that was so far favorable to the company ("Conference of Pharmaceutical Department," 28 May 1913, BAL). He appears to be ignoring the numerous criticisms that had already appeared in the pages of *JAMA* leveled against Bayer's use of patents and trade names. See also James Burrow, *Organized Medicine in the Progressive Era: The Move toward Monopoly* (Baltimore: Johns Hopkins University Press, 1977); Jan R. McTavish, "'What's in a Name?' Aspirin and the American Medical Association," *Bulletin of the History of Medicine* 61 (1987): 342–366.

13.   The dearth of raw materials from Germany sent Bayer's prices up, but Aspirin continued to be advertised throughout the war. In 1916, Aspirin cost eighty-five cents per ounce wholesale, and phenacetin was $2.15. By early 1918, Aspirin was still eighty-five cents but phenacetin was now $3.50.

14.   "Big Campaign for Aspirin to Forestall Expiration of Patents," *Printers Ink* 95 (1916): 189–191.

15.   The ads did not appear, however, in the *New York Tribune* at this time.

16.   "Aspirin," *JAMA* 68l (1917): 213.

17.   "Acetylsalicylic Acid, Not Aspirin," *JAMA* 68 (1917): 201–202.

18.   *Philadelphia Public Ledger*, 10 February, 1917, p. 15, col. 3; Carroll Hochwalt, "The Story of Aspirin," *Chemistry* 301 (1957): 10–14; "Defense of Monsanto Chemical Works in Suit over 'Aspirin' Trade-Mark," *Drug and Chemical Markets* 4 (1917–1918): 8. See also Dan J. Forrestal, *Faith, Hope and $5,000: The Story of Monsanto—The Trials and Triumphs of the First Seventy-five Years* (New York: Simon and Schuster, 1977), chap. 1.

19.   "Acetylsalicylic Acid, or 'What's in a Name?'" *JAMA* 70 (1918): 1097. Quality was a problem, however. Not all American-made ASA was as good as the original. See Robert C. White, "The Manufacture of Aspirin Tablets," *American Journal of Pharmacy* 90 (1918): 640–646.

20.   *CARD News*, February 1917, 2. "Bayer and Co. Threaten Aspirin Suits. Will Defend Patent Rights in Court if Necessary. Effect of Advertising Campaign," *Pharmaceutical Era* 49 (1916): 402.

21.   Advertisement in *Deutsch Amerikanische-Apotheker Zeitung* 38 (1917–1918).

22.   See Mann and Plummer, *Aspirin Wars*, 66. An advertisement for Liggett's (i.e., Rexall) drugstores in New York City, appearing in the *New York Times*, 6 June 1916, p. 6, listed "Aspirin Tablets" at twenty-four for thirty-five cents, and one hundred for $1.10, but it does not describe these as Bayer's product, although if they were not Bayer they infringed on the patent. The first Bayer newspaper advertisements appeared the following month.

23.   "Aspirin and the Drug Trade," *Bulletin of Pharmacy* 31 (March 1917): 84.

24.   Williams Haynes, *The American Chemical Industry: A History*, 6 vols. (New York: Van Nostrand, 1945–1954), 3:315; Charles LaWall, "The Supply of Pharmaceuticals

and Medicines in War Time; Its Importance and Dangers," *American Journal of Public Health* 9 (1919): 181–183; U.S. Government, *Reports of the Alien Property Custodian, 1918–1919* (Washington, D.C.: Government Printing Office, 1919), chaps. 1 and 2; Mann and Plummer, *Aspirin Wars*, 44ff.

25. "Dr. Hugo Schweitzer Dies," *New York Times*, 24 December 1917, p. 9, col. 8; "Memorial Service for Dr. Schweitzer," *New York Times*, 30 December 1917, sec. 1, p. 15, col. 1; "Dr. Schweitzer Memorial Not Held," *Drug and Chemical Markets* 4 (1917–1918): 32. Later, there were rumors that Schweitzer was hiding in Mexico, but these were total fabrications. APC, RG 131, entry 199, case file 4062, box 159, National Archives. Also see "Aspirin and Espionage," *JAMA* 72 (1919): 740.

26. U.S. House of Representatives, Committee on Ways and Means, *Dyestuffs* (Washington, D.C.: Government Printing Office, 1919), 139.

27. One of Germany's alleged agents fell asleep on the New York subway. "Waking up at his stop, he rushed out of the train, leaving behind a briefcase full of secret papers," which was promptly picked up by an American Secret Service agent (Mann and Plummer, *Aspirin Wars*, 41). But also see the "authorized history" of the American Protective League, which credits the Germans with greater efficiency: Emerson Hough, *The Web* (Chicago: Reilly and Lee, 1919). In addition, see Ellen Janet Jenkins, "Organizing Victory: Great Britain, The United States and the Instruments of War, 1914–1916," Ph.D. dissertation, University of North Texas, 1992, chap. 8; Jules Witcover, *Sabotage at Black Tom: Imperial Germany's Secret War in America, 1914–1917* (Chapel Hill, N.C.: Algonquin Books, 1989). Witcover does not mention the Bayer Company's alleged involvement in the spy business, even as a rumor.

28. See Mann and Plummer, *Aspirin Wars*, 39–42. Schweitzer's salary from Bayer was about $12,000 per year. At his death, his account in the German American Bank had a balance of $1,478,882.08. APC, RG 131, entry 199, case file 4062, box 159, National Archives.

29. Reimer, "Bayer," 196–236.

30. "What's in a Name?" *Journal of Industrial and Engineering Chemistry* 10 (1918): 255.

31. Advertisement in *Deutsch Amerikanische-Apotheker Zeitung* 38 (August 1917): 75; advertisement in *Medical Times* 46 (October 1918).

32. Garner's Drug Store, Tulsa, Okla., to A. Mitchell Palmer, 6 August 1918, APC, RG 131, entry 155, CM 201, box 35, National Archives.

33. Kimball and Stone, druggists, Bakersfield, to Alien Property Custodian, 19 September 1918, APC, RG 131, entry 155, CM 201, box 35, National Archives.

34. National Association of Retail Druggists to A. Mitchell Palmer, 21 August 1918, APC, RG 131, entry 155, CM 201, box 35, National Archives.

35. H. Schmidt, "America's Financial Contribution to Germany on Account of Our Patent Laws," *JAMA* 68 (1917): 1648. He said the English paid six cents an ounce for aspirin, while Americans paid thirty-seven cents.

36. John Bowker, Lawrence, Mass., to A. Mitchell Palmer, 14 April 1918, APC, RG 131, entry 155, CM 201, box 35, National Archives. The earlier letter is not in the file.

37. Corporate Management Division to the Frederick Pharmacy, Huntington, W. Va., 17 October 1918, APC, RG 131, entry 155, CM 201, box 35, National Archives.

38. Alien Property Custodian to Howard Crawley, Washington, D.C., 5 September 1918, APC, RG 131, entry 155, CM 201, box 35, National Archives. This letter was in response to Mr. Crawley's complaint of 1 September that Bayer was masquerading as an American firm.

39. Charles Herty, editor of the *Journal of Industrial and Engineering Chemistry*, to A. Mitchell Palmer, 14 October 1918, APC, RG 131, entry 155, CM 201, box 35, National Archives.

40. Letter from the Frederick Pharmacy, Huntington, W. Va., 12 October 1918, APC, RG 131, entry 155, CM 201, box 35, National Archives.

41. Photostat of letter, L. Ruby Reid, American Red Cross, Wake Forest Branch, N.C., to the Department of Justice, 14 October 1918, APC, RG 131, entry 155, CM 201, box 35, National Archives.

42. On Sunday, 14 April 1918, the last page of the first rotogravure section of the *New York Times* featured a full-page illustration of the Bayer factory at Rensselaer, informing New Yorkers that Aspirin had been "Made on the Banks of the Hudson River" since 1904. There was also an exhortation for "every loyal American to buy Liberty Bonds and War Savings Stamps."

43. Investigator's report, "In Re: Bayer's Aspirin Tablets, Alleged German Plot to Spread Spanish Influenza," New Orleans, 31 October 1918, APC, RG 131, entry 199, file 1048, box 43, National Archives.

44. Letter from Edward Heath Peters, 14 October 1918, APC, RG 131, entry 155, CM 201, box 35, National Archives.

45. C. G. Trumbull, editor of the *Sunday School Times* (Philadelphia), to A. Mitchell Palmer, 3 October 1918, APC, RG 131, entry 155, CM 201, box 35, National Archives.

46. Mrs. Moulton Green to the Committee on Public Information, 18 August 1918, APC, RG 131, entry 155, CM 201, box 35, National Archives.

47. Report of the investigator, New York City, 6 April 1918. He interviewed the advertising agency and was satisfied that secret messages were not being sent. The intelligence officer in question, however, had been suspicious months earlier. Letter to B. Bielaski, Department of Justice, 29 August 1917, APC, RG 131, entry 199, file 1048, box 43, National Archives.

48. The investigators' reports indicate that apparently they tried first to determine if any part of the rumors was true, and second, to learn how the rumors were being spread. APC, RG 131, entry 199, file 1048, box 43, National Archives.

49. Profits totaled more than $672,000, but of this, $400,000 went to Synthetic Patents and $130,000 was reserved for Farbenfabriken in Germany. Records of

the Bureau of Audits [WWI], In re: Examination of the Books of Seized Companies, box 3, Bayer Company, APC, RG 131, entry 134, National Archives.

50. Transcript of Senate Hearings concerning the alleged dye monopoly, 2 March
1922, p. 960, APC, RG 131, entry 14, National Archives.

51. Letter from C. H. Morgan, M.D., 10 September 1918; pharmacist Emil Backer,
New Ulm, Minn., to the Bayer Company, 9 September 1918; both in APC, RG 131,
entry 155, CM 201, box 35, National Archives.

52. Mann and Plummer, *Aspirin Wars*, 50–80. In the years following the Great War,
the German chemical industry was suspected of engaging in innumerable illegal or questionable activities, not least of which was helping Germany get ready
for another world war. The giant Interessengemeinschaft der Farbenindustrie
Aktiengesellschaft (IG Farben) that was formed in 1925, and included both Bayer
and Hoechst, was a formidable cartel that after 1933 was closely associated with
the Nazis. See Victor Lefebure, *The Riddle of the Rhine: Chemical Strategy in Peace
and War* (New York: Chemical Foundation, 1923); Howard Ambruster, *Treason's
Peace: German Dyes and American Dupes* (New York: Beechurst, 1947); Josiah R.
Dubois, Jr., *The Devil's Chemists: Twenty-four Years of the International Farben Cartel Who Manufacture Wars* (Boston: Beacon Press, 1952); Peter Hayes, *Industry and
Ideology: IG Farben in the Nazi Era* (Cambridge: Cambridge University Press, 1987).
Hayes is more sympathetic to IG Farben than are the other authors and does not
support the view that the IG was simply a Nazi front.

53. "Proprieties in Advertising," *American Journal of Pharmacy* 91 (1919): 489–493.

54. "The CPA Winnipeg Convention," *Canadian Pharmaceutical Journal* 53 (1919):
103–104. Quotations are from "Druggists to Fight German Aggression," 9 October 1919, *Winnipeg Free Press*, p. 1. col. 3. Although at this particular moment
Sterling had struck no deals with German Bayer, by 1923 Aspirin in Canada
would be far more German than was Aspirin in the United States, in that Sterling agreed to pay German Bayer 50 percent of the profits from the sale of Bayer
Aspirin in Canada. This agreement remained in effect even through World War
II ("Amerika-Besprechung," 9 April 1923, 4/C. 34.5, BAL).

55. Haynes, *American Chemical Industry*, 6:407; *Poor's Manual of Industrials: Manufacturing, Mining, and Miscellaneous Companies*, 9th annual (New York: Poor's Manual Co., 1918), 2142.

56. Miscellaneous Products, Miscellaneous Advertisements, 1914–1948, box 510,
Sterling Incorporated Archives, History Factory, Chantilly, Va. These headache
powders were in fact among the very few whose ads can sometimes be found in
pre-war American newspapers.

57. Product Files, Domestic Advertisements, 1923–1930, box 419, Sterling Incorporated Archives.

58. Ibid.

59. Resolution of the Committee on Standardization, 1915, Executive Committee minutes, Proprietary Association of America, CHPA, Washington, D.C.

60. "Aspirin-Bayer and the Sterling Products Company," *JAMA* 76 (1921): 1697.

61. F. B. Young, "Ill-Advised References to Treatment in Articles on Public Health Problems," *JAMA* 71 (1918): 1337.

62. Advertisements—Domestic, 1918–1922, box 406, Sterling Incorporated Archives.

63. Roger Lee, *The Happy Life of a Doctor* (Boston: Little, Brown, 1956), 194.

64. N. S. Yawger, "Indurative Headache," *JAMA* 52 (1909): 1316–1319. Yawger treated this rheumatic condition with many different salicylates, including Aspirin. As a sufferer, he had also tried the regimen on himself and could vouch for its effectiveness.

65. Milwaukee drugstore prescription files, file C39q, Kremers Reference Files, University of Wisconsin, Madison.

66. See E. N. Gathercoal, *The Prescription Ingredient Survey* (Chicago: APhA, 1933), 28.

67. A.R.L. Dohme, "Report of the Sub-Committee on Acetylsalicylic Acid," *Proceedings of the American Drug Manufacturers Association* 8 (1919): 234–235.

68. Farbenfabriken vorm. Fr. Bayer und Co., "Aspirin," in *Pharmazeutische Produkt* (Elberfeld: Bayer, 1906), 76.

69. J. Lindsay and A. J. Bruce Leckie, letter to the editor, *British Medical Journal* 1 (1913): 1108.

70. Lee, *Happy Life*, 194. See also Julian Loudon, "Headaches Due to Disease of the Nervous System," *Canadian Practitioner* 39 (1914): 702–706; Samuel Salinger, "Treatment of Sick Headache," *New York Medical Journal* 88 (1908): 1037–1038; W. J. Wilson, "Headaches Due to Deranged Metabolism," *Canadian Practitioner* 39 (1914): 697–699.

71. Wesley Taylor, "Headache," *New York Medical Journal* 94 (1911): 674–678.

72. Nestor Tirard, "Some Clinical Observations with New Remedies," *Lancet* 1 (1905): 83–84.

73. "Aspirin," *JAMA* 68 (1917): 213.

74. Although the diagnoses were not mentioned, a survey in 1909 found that phenacetin was prescribed more than four million times that year in the United States, in a population of about 90 million (Gathercoal, *Prescription Survey*, 21).

75. Even after Bayer's product was deleted, the *NNR* retained ASA, but this sentence appeared in every edition from at least 1915 until 1949, when ASA was no longer considered for inclusion. It is clear evidence that Aspirin had been a headache treatment well in advance of public advertising.

76. "The Aspirin Trade-Mark," *Chemist and Druggist* 86 (1915): 16–17, 79.

77. The organic chemical industry in the United States had often complained that the German way of doing business prevented a native industry from thriving, and it took every opportunity provided by the war and its aftermath to demon-

strate both competence and superiority. In 1918, all samples but one of American ASA were considered equal to Bayer's. P. N. Leech, "Examination of American-Made Acetylsalicylic Acid," *Journal of Industrial and Engineering Chemistry* 10 (1918): 288–290. Consequently, many manufacturers were poised to provide high-quality, home-grown synthetic drugs at competitive prices even before the war ended. In addition to Haynes, *American Chemical Industry*, vol. 3, see Alfred S. Burdick, "The Manufacture of Synthetic Medicinal Chemicals in America," *Journal of the American Pharmaceutical Association* 11 (1922): 98–108; Maurice L. Tainter and G. M. A. Marcelli, "The Rise of Synthetic Drugs in the American Pharmaceutical Industry," *Bulletin of the New York Academy of Medicine* 35 (1959): 387–405. The antipathy to the German companies, however, has tended to skew the historical view of them. Thomas Reimer attempts to set the record straight ("Bayer," chap. 6).

78. "Aspirin Held Not to Be a Trade-Mark," *Druggists Circular* 63 (1919): 36.

79. Mann and Plummer, *Aspirin Wars*, 46.

80. "The Aspirin Decision," *Drug and Chemical Markets* 8 (1921): 984.

81. "Aspirin or Acetylsalicylic Acid—An Important Court Decision," *JAMA* 76 (1921): 1356.

82. Anonymous typescript, untitled, incomplete, ca. 1942, reporting on Sterling's association with IG Farben, file C38 (a)I, Sterling Drug Company, Kremers Reference Files.

83. The red band was truly red, and the full-color trade ads could not have been missed. Like Bayer, Smith, Kline and French offered counter displays of "Tin Box Twelves" that "Go Like Hot Cakes. Put this display case on your counter and Watch 'Em Sell." They exhorted druggists to "Advertise an Aspirin that *Pays.*" They also noted that Smith, Kline and French provided "*Genuine Aspirin*, made by Americans, and backed by three-quarters of a century's drug experience"; *NARD Journal* 29 (1919).

84. Paul Olsen, *The Merchandising of Drug Products* (New York: D. Appleton-Century, 1931), 47.

85. Advertisement in *Practical Druggist*, November 1934. Most non-Bayer aspirin seems to have been advertised publicly only in newspaper drugstore ads.

86. Mann and Plummer, *Aspirin Wars*, 156.

87. *Albuquerque Journal*, 12 June 1936.

88. "The unit is small and fifteen cents will buy the highest priced one in any store. Therefore, this business goes to the better known manufacturers without much of a struggle"; "Aspirin," *Drug and Cosmetic Industry* 35 (1935): 275–276.

89. "But when the consumer goes into the drug store to buy a bottle of 100 tablets for the medicine chest, . . . [he is] much more likely to be swayed by the lower prices of the less known brands. This accounts for the fact that the less known brands sell such a high proportion of bottles" (ibid.). The growth of drugstore chains (523 chains with 4,053 stores by 1931) fostered the spread of house

brands and actually reduced the sales of branded items. William J. Baxter, *Chain Store Distribution and Management* (New York: Harper and Brothers, 1931), 5, 314.

90. "Aspirin," *Drug and Cosmetic Industry* 43 (1938): 27. In 1933, more than 3.1 million pounds had been sold. Besides being useful for treating pain, aspirin, it was rumored, taken together with Coca-Cola, produced a cheap "high" that during Prohibition was also legal. See Mark Pendergrast, *For God, Country, and Coca-Cola: The Unauthorized History of the Great American Soft-Drink and the Company That Makes It* (New York: Scribners, 1993), 191.

91. John W. Shurman, "A Case of Chronic Acetanilidism," *JAMA* 77 (1921): 526; William Reid, "The Heart in Acetphenetidin Poisoning," *JAMA* 87 (1926): 1036–1037.

92. James Walsh, "Forty-five Years of Personal Experience with Headache," *International Clinics* 3 (1930): 135–147. He also never apparently realized that Antikamnia started out as acetanilid and then became acetphenetidin as a result of the 1906 law.

93. "An-A-Cin," *JAMA* 92 (1929): 1881. See also "Anacin: The Birth and Development of a 'Patent Medicine,'" *JAMA* 85 (1925): 1079.

94. Mann and Plummer, *Aspirin Wars*, 154–160; Haynes, *American Chemical Industry*, 6:26–30.

95. In the convoluted present-day world of drug company mergers and takeovers, Alka-Seltzer, once the property of Miles Laboratories of Elkhart, Ind., is now owned by Bayer AG of Leverkusen. Moreover, Bayer as it exists today in America is the German company again, Sterling having been bought first by Kodak in 1988, sold to SmithKline Beecham in August 1994, and then immediately sold to Bayer AG in September 1994.

96. The older drugs still had their champions. One acetanilid manufacturer, for example, produced a series of advertisements for pharmaceutical journals, quoting authorities who called "acetanilid . . . by far the most powerful antineuralgic at our disposal" and urging its continued use in domestic and professional practice. Advertisement in *American Druggist* 91 (1935): 22 (February). This ad is headed with a notice: "No. 13 of a Series of Advertisements Presented in the Interest of Acetanilid U.S.P. by the Emerson Drug Company." There were at least twenty-three of these ads and possibly more. They do not seem to single out headache, but Emerson's Bromo-Seltzer did, at least as illustrated by its prewar advertising: a big blue bottle, with a white label and large blue lettering proclaimed "Emerson's Bromo-Seltzer Cures Headaches."

97. Arthur J. Cramp, "Truth in Advertising Drug Products," *American Journal of Public Health* 10 (1920): 783–789.

98. Arthur J. Cramp, "Headaches and 'Aspirin,'" *Hygeia* 1 (1923): 316–317. See also "Concerning a Favorite Drug," *American Review of Reviews* 68 (1923): 661–662, which likewise advised caution. On *Hygeia* itself, see Morris Fishbein, *A History of the American Medical Association, 1847–1947* (Philadelphia: W. B. Saunders,

1947), 272, 320, 325, 1185. For reasons Fishbein does not explain, the AMA exec-
utives at first were reluctant to approve the magazine.

99. There were further dangers from self-treatment in that the drugs could be mis-
branded or adulterated. Solon R. Barber, "Headache Relief," *Hygeia* 10 (1932):
226–228. This was presumed to be less likely to happen if the drugs were
obtained by prescription.

100. "Comparative Value of Acetylsalicylic Acid and Acetanilid as Analgesics," *JAMA*
73 (1919): 1383–1384. The costs were similar but ASA was deemed less toxic.

101. T. Swann Harding, *Fads, Frauds, and Physicians: Diagnosis and Treatment of the Doctors' Dilemma* (New York: Dial Press, 1930), 173.

102. "If you value your health, beware of the aspirin habit." R. L. Alsaker, *Headaches:
Cause, Prevention, and Cure* (New York: Frank E. Morrison, 1919), 53. Two physicians from Pennsylvania observed a man with tuberculosis of the neck who took
fifteen hundred grains of aspirin a week (about three hundred tablets); even
after a stay in the hospital he still craved the drug. These authors did not note
any damage to this patient (not even gastric upset) and were in fact concerned
only that he had become addicted. J. Allen Jackson and Horace V. Pike, "Aspirin
Addiction—Report of a Case Using 1500 Grains Weekly," *Therapeutic Gazette* 46
(1922): 692–693.

103. Cramp, "Headaches and 'Aspirin.' " See also "Concerning a Favorite Drug."

104. "Headache Medicines," *Hygeia* 5 (1927): 320; "Aspirins," *Hygeia* 7 (1929): 830;
"Acetylsalicylic Acid," *JAMA* 80 (1923): 1092.

105. "Dangers of Large Doses of Acetylsalicylic Acid," *JAMA* 91 (1928): 344.

106. Arthur Kallet and F. J. Schlink, *100,000,000 Guinea Pigs* (New York: Grossett and
Dunlap, 1933), 71–72. This book was in its thirty-second printing by 1937. See
James Harvey Young, "Social History of American Drug Legislation," in *Drugs in
Our Society*, ed. Paul Talalay (Baltimore: Johns Hopkins University Press, 1964),
226. The problem of allergic reactions was exemplified by a case from India, in
which a planter, knowing he could not take aspirin, took Empirin instead.
Empirin was merely a British brand name for ASA. "Case of Intolerance to
Aspirin," *Therapeutic Gazette* 45 (1921): 492.

107. Harold Aaron, "Alka-Seltzer: The Medical View," *Consumer Reports* 1 (May 1936):
6–7.

108. "A Blacklist of Drugs and Cosmetics," *Consumer Reports* 2 (August 1936): 22–23.

109. Mann and Plummer, *Aspirin Wars*, 138–150.

110. "Colds," *Consumer Reports* 2 (January–February 1937): 12–16.

111. On the FDA and its activities in this period, see Charles Jackson, *Food and Drug
Legislation in the New Deal* (Princeton: Princeton University Press, 1970); Gwen
Kay, "Healthy Public Relations: The FDA's 1930s Legislative Campaign," *Bulletin
of the History of Medicine* 75 (2001): 446–487.

112. James Burrow, *AMA: Voice of American Medicine* (Baltimore: Johns Hopkins University Press, 1963), 252.

113. Peter Temin, *Taking Your Medicine: Drug Regulation in the United States* (Cambridge: Harvard University Press, 1980), 41.

114. Sulfanilamide was hailed as a wonder drug when it was introduced as Prontosil in 1935 by Bayer (now part of IG Farben) because it was particularly effective against streptococcal infections. But its trademark and patent resurrected criticism of Bayer's practices.

115. Jackson, *Food and Drug Legislation*, 151–154.

116. A brief summary of the law's provisions can be found in James Harvey Young, "Federal Drug and Narcotic Legislation," *Pharmacy in History* 37 (1995): 59–65. A more detailed account, from which I have drawn my remarks, is in Temin, *Taking Your Medicine*, 38–57.

117. Temin, *Taking Your Medicine*, 38–51; quotation, 47.

118. James Harvey Young, *The Medical Messiahs: A Social History of Health Quackery in Twentieth-Century America* (Princeton: Princeton University Press, 1967), 297.

119. Mann and Plummer (*Aspirin Wars*, 138–150) describe the situation in some detail and note that the drug industry treated the 1938 law "as a victory."

120. "Something for a Headache," *Hygeia* 2 (1924): 374.

121. Francis W. Palfrey, "Headache," *Hygeia* 7 (1929): 238–241. See also Solon R. Barber, "Headache Relief," 226–228, which reiterated the need to seek causes.

CHAPTER 8   THE HEADACHE IN THE TWENTIETH CENTURY

1. Eben J. Carey, *Medical Science Exhibits, A Century of Progress: Chicago World's Fair, 1933 and 1934* (Chicago, 1936), 25.

2. Roy Porter, *The Greatest Benefit to Mankind* (New York: W. W. Norton, 1997), 601.

3. This was the general feeling of Francis W. Peabody, *Doctor and Patient: Papers on the Relationship of the Physician to Men and Institutions* (New York: Macmillan, 1930).

4. Paul Starr, *The Social Transformation of American Medicine: The Rise of a Sovereign Profession and the Making of a Vast Industry* (New York: Basic Books, 1982), 127; John Burnham notes that in the first fifty years of the twentieth century, the medical profession suffered less criticism than in any other period before or since. He describes the "priestly functions" that physicians assumed and the high expectations of both the profession and the public. John C. Burnham, "American Medicine's Golden Age: What Happened to It?" *Science* 215 (1982): 1474–1479.

5. Robert A. Buerki, "American Pharmaceutical Education, 1902–1952," *Journal of the American Pharmaceutical Association* 41 (2001): 519–521.

6. For a brief outline of the ethical manufacturers' organizations, see Dennis B.

Worthen, "The Pharmaceutical Industry, 1902–1952," *Journal of the American Pharmaceutical Association* 41 (2001): 656–659.

7. See the various works by John P. Swann, "The Evolution of the American Pharmaceutical Industry," *Pharmacy in History* 37 (1995): 76–86; *Academic Scientists and the Pharmaceutical Industry: Cooperative Research in Twentieth-Century America* (Baltimore: Johns Hopkins University Press, 1988); "Insulin: A Case Study in the Emergence of Collaborative Pharmaceutical Research," *Pharmacy in History* 28 (1986): 3–13, 65–74; "Institutional Frameworks for Drug Research in America, *Pharmacy in History* 32 (1990): 3–11. See also Ernst Chain, "Academic and Industrial Contributions to Drug Research," *Nature* 200 (1963): 441–451; John Parascandola, "Industrial Research Comes of Age: The American Pharmaceutical Industry, 1920–1940," *Pharmacy in History* 27 (1985): 12–21.

8. Jay S. Cohen, *Over Dose: The Case against the Drug Companies: Prescription Drugs, Side Effects and Your Health* (New York: Jeremy P. Tarcher, 2001), 147–151. Cohen discusses a great many of the problems he sees not so much in the products themselves but in the way they are marketed. See also Marcia Angell, "The Pharmaceutical Industry—To Whom Is It Accountable?" *New England Journal of Medicine* 342 (2000): 1902–1904. But these are simply among the latest critiques of the drug trade. In addition to those already mentioned in chap. 3, n. 17, see Jerry Avorn, Milton Chen, and Robert Hartley, "Scientific versus Commercial Sources of Influence on the Prescribing Behavior of Physicians," *American Journal of Medicine* 73 (1982): 4–8. The manager of domestic sales for Schering Corporation provided a guidebook: Arthur Peterson, *Pharmaceutical Selling, "Detailing," and Sales Training* (New York: McGraw-Hill, 1949).

9. In addition to Starr, *Social Transformation of American Medicine,* see Elton Rayack, *Professional Power and American Medicine: The Economics of the American Medical Association* (Cleveland: World Publishing, 1967). Rayack discusses the difference between restricting a profession in order to control the market versus controlling a profession in order to improve services.

10. British scientist John Vane received the 1982 Nobel Prize in medicine for his work in unraveling how aspirin actually works as an analgesic (by inhibiting the production of prostaglandins), but I am not aware of any practical application of this knowledge in headache treatment.

11. Robert T. Stormont, "A Physician Looks at Proprietary Drugs," *Drug and Cosmetic Industry* 71 (1952): 471.

12. Lord Dawson of Penn, "Some Varieties of Headache," *British Medical Journal* 2 (1927): 607–609, 652.

13. Stewart Tepper, "From Moldy Bread to DHE: A History of the Ergot Drugs," *Headache the Newsletter of ACHE* 8 (1997).

14. A short account of Wolff and his work is in Donald J. Dalessio, "Remembrances of Dr. Harold G. Wolff," in *Wolff's "Headache and Other Head Pain,"* 7th ed., ed.

Stephen D. Silberstein, Richard B. Lipton, and Donald J. Dalessio (New York: Oxford University Press, 2001).

15. That aspirin is in fact better than placebo was confirmed by various studies. See John H. Beckley and Erwin Di Cyan, "Popular Headache Remedies," *Headache* 1 (April 1961): 25–27; William J. Murray, "Evaluation of Aspirin in Treatment of Headache," *Clinical Pharmacology and Therapeutics* 5 (1964): 21–25.

16. For an excellent account of the problem of pain in American medicine, see Mary S. Sheridan, *Pain in America* (Tuscaloosa: University of Alabama Press, 1992). Also see Helen Neal, *The Politics of Pain* (New York: McGraw-Hill, 1978). On the impact of the Harrison Narcotic Act, see Edward M. Brecher, *Licit and Illicit Drugs* (Boston: Little, Brown, 1972), 48–55, as well as material in H. Wayne Morgan, *Drugs in America: A Social History, 1800–1980* (Syracuse, N.Y.: Syracuse University Press, 1981); David F. Musto, *The American Disease: Origins of Narcotics Control*, 2nd ed. (New York: Oxford University Press, 1987); David Courtwright, *Dark Paradise: Opiate Addiction in America before 1940* (Cambridge: Harvard University Press, 1982).

17. The first quotation is attributed to J. Sadger, as referred to in *Psychoanalytic Review* 1 (1913–1914): 230. For an account of Freud's view of headaches, see A. Karwautz, C. Wöber-Bingöl, and C. Wöber, "Freud and Migraine: The Beginning of a Psychodynamically Oriented View of Headache a Hundred Years Ago," *Cephalalgia* 16 (1996): 22–26. The second quotation is from Jule Eisenbud, "The Psychology of Headache: A Case Studied Experimentally," *Psychiatric Quarterly* 11 (1937): 592–619.

18. See Charles S. Adler, Sheila M. Adler, and Arnold Friedman, "A Historical Perspective on Psychiatric Thinking about Headache," in *Psychiatric Aspects of Headache*, ed. Charles S. Adler, Sheila M. Adler, and Russell C. Packard (Baltimore: Williams and Wilkins, 1987).

19. J. Lincoln McCartney, "Psychogenic Headaches with the Treatment of a Case," *National Medical Journal of China* 12 (1925–1926): 359–371; J. Lincoln McCartney, "Headaches: With Special Reference to those of Psychogenic Origin," *China Medical Journal* 39 (1925): 32–40.

20. *Psychosomatic Medicine* 2 (1940), referring to an article by Frieda Fromm-Reichmann in *Psychoanalytic Review* 24 (1937): 26–112.

21. Jay H. Schmidt, "Deep Hostility, the Nose and Headache," *Headache* 3 (April 1963): 32–34.

22. Louis G. Moench, *Headache*, 2nd ed. (Chicago: Yearbook Publishers, 1951), 199.

23. Harold G. Wolff, "Personality Features and Reactions of Subjects with Migraines," *Archives of Neurology and Psychiatry* 37 (1937): 895–921.

24. Robert Marcussen and Harold G. Wolff, "A Formulation of the Dynamics of the Migraine Attack," *Psychosomatic Medicine* 11 (1949): 251–256.

25. Walter C. Alvarez, *Help Your Doctor to Help You When You Have a Sick Headache or Migraine* (New York: Harper and Brothers, 1941), 1–20.

26. Marcussen and Wolff, "Dynamics of Migraine," 255.

27. Robert Ryan, *Headache: Diagnosis and Treatment* (St. Louis: C. V. Mosby, 1954), chap. 13, on psychogenic headache; quotations on pp. 117–128.

28. Noah Fabricant, *Headache: What Causes Them, How to Get Relief* (New York: Farrar, Straus, 1949), 82. The failure to recognize psychological elements was in large part the doctor's fault. See Arnold Friedman, *Modern Headache Therapy* (St. Louis: C. V. Mosby, 1951), 128, in which he complains about the "tardy application of psychiatric knowledge to the problems of general practice."

29. Hugh Garland, ed., *Medicine*, 2 vols. (London: Macmillan, 1953), 1:277–280; Seymour Diamond and William B. Furlong, *More Than Two Aspirin: Hope for Your Headache Problem* (Chicago: Follett, 1976), 247.

30. Frederick Tilney, "Etiological Considerations of Headache," *Bulletin of the New York Academy of Medicine* 11 (1935): 500–510. Twenty years later, another physician noted of his tension headache patients: "I must say that many of my patients do not appear to have any present problem which can be defined as unresolved conflict. They simply have a habit of muscular contraction which has been with them through an otherwise untroubled life." James Lance, *Headache: Understanding, Alleviation* (New York: Scribners' Sons, 1975), 110–111. See also "Psychosomatic Research," *Journal of Psychosomatic Research* 1 (1956): 1. The inaugural volume lamented that the psychosomatic approach "suffers from a surfeit of unverified and inadequately validated hypotheses and a paucity of established facts." To gain credibility, the field needed better standards.

31. Ryan, *Headache*, 124–126. A dramatic example of how a personality change could cure headaches was described by Marcussen and Wolff ("Dynamics of Migraine," 254) in a male patient whose previously undetected syphilis finally became apparent. Paradoxically, his migraines ceased. The "syphilis caused a change in personality structure. . . . The disorganization of his personality was such to prevent the development of the pernicious cycle which had previously led to headache."

32. Moench, *Headache*, 205–206.

33. Charles Brenner, Arnold Friedman, and Sidney Carter, "Psychologic Factors in the Etiology and Treatment of Chronic Headache," *Psychosomatic Medicine* 11 (1949): 53–56.

34. Harold G. Wolff, *Headache and Other Head Pain* (New York: Oxford University Press, 1948).

35. As always, the variety of headache types and the subjectivity of the pain experience made them difficult to study. In 1988 the International Headache Society (established in Great Britain in 1981) proposed a classification scheme that is now the accepted standard. It provides guidance in assessing patients and a means to evaluate the effects of therapy. This system has thirteen major categories, including migraine, tension-type, cluster (a particularly vicious series of headaches that affects men more than women), headaches associated with head trauma, with ears, sinuses, and the teeth, and those associated with metabolic disorders, along

with "headache not classifiable," and several subcategories such as "cluster headache–like disorder not fulfilling above criteria." On some level this system of classification does not appear to be altogether different from its century-old predecessors—except for the notable absence of constipation as a cause.

36. Stephen D. Silberstein, Richard B. Lipton, and Peter J. Goadsby, *Headache in Clinical Practice* (London and New York: Martin Dunitz, 2002), 113. Silberstein, by the way, works at the Jefferson Headache Center, Thomas Jefferson University, Philadelphia. One wonders what Jefferson himself might have thought of this.

37. J. B. Spooner and J. G. Harvey, "The History and Usage of Paracetamol [Acetaminophen] Winthrop," *Journal of International Medical Research* 4 (1976): suppl. 4, 1–6. Acetaminophen in large doses can harm the liver. For an account of the other remedies, see Charles Mann and Mark L. Plummer, *The Aspirin Wars: Money, Medicine, and One Hundred Years of Rampant Competition* (New York: Alfred A. Knopf, 1991).

38. "Too many patients have left physicians' offices with the message that 'nothing serious is the matter' and they 'have to learn to live with headaches,' so they give up hope of appropriate treatment and relief of pain." Alan M. Rapoport and Fred D. Sheftell, *Headache Disorders: A Management Guide for the Practitioner* (Philadelphia: W. B. Saunders, 1996), vii.

INDEX

ABOUT THE AUTHOR

Jan R. McTavish holds a Ph.D. in history and history of science from York University in Toronto and has taught at the University of Winnipeg, the University of California Los Angeles, and Alcorn State University.